lots of pleasure
with this

Ace
xxx

BISEXUALITY

&

HIV/AIDS

New Concepts in Human Sexuality Series

Vern L. Bullough, Series Editor

BISEXUALITY
&
HIV/AIDS

A Global Perspective

edited by
Rob Tielman
Manuel Carballo
Aart Hendriks

PROMETHEUS BOOKS ■ BUFFALO, NEW YORK

Published 1991 by Prometheus Books

95 94 93 92 91   5 4 3 2 1

Library of Congress Cataloging-in-Publication Data

Bisexuality and HIV/AIDS : a global perspective / edited by Rob A. P. Tielman, Manuel Carballo, and Aart C. Hendriks.
     p.   cm.—(New concepts in human sexuality)
  Includes bibliographical references and index.
  ISBN 0-87975-666-7 (cloth : alk. paper)
  1. AIDS (Disease)—Epidemiology. 2. Bisexuality. I. Tielman, Rob, 1946-   . II. Carballo, Manuel, 1941-   . III. Hendriks, Aart C. IV. Series.
RA644.A25B57   1991
616.97'92'008663—dc20   91-16625
                                                 CIP

Printed in the United States of America on acid-free paper.

Contents

6   Contents

PART 2: A THEMATIC SURVEY OF BISEXUALITY AND HIV/AIDS

Preface

Thanks to the initiative and the support of the Global Programme on AIDS (GPA) of the World Health Organization (WHO), the Gay and Lesbian Studies Department of the University of Utrecht in the Netherlands was able to bring together this anthology. The contributors enthusiastically accepted the invitation to participate in the first published inventory of the pattern of bisexuality and HIV/AIDS, based upon a number of strict principles and goals. Their conclusions are based mainly upon data obtained by existing studies and may thus be said to reflect the current state of knowledge about the interrelationship of bisexuality and HIV/AIDS.

We, the editors, are grateful for the willingness of the authors to collaborate in this challenging project, which became known as the "bisexuality book." As editors, we had the advantage of becoming familiar with the important studies being undertaken by these highly committed persons, often with very limited resources. On behalf of the contributors, we want to express our hope that this anthology will contribute to developing effective and accurate health intervention strategies to prevent further HIV transmission and eventually to combat AIDS, in full respect of basic human rights and freedoms, notably the right to individual self-determination.

Our involvement with the bisexuality and HIV/AIDS topic does not end with the publication of this book. In the meantime, all necessary preparations have been made to conduct worldwide cross-cultural qualitative research into this field. This research project will be coordinated by the Gay and Lesbian Studies Department, with the financial support of the World Health Organization's Global Programme on AIDS and the Dutch Government.

Utrecht/Geneva, February 1991

Prof. Dr. Rob A. P. Tielman
Manuel Carballo, Ph.D.
Aart C. Hendriks, LL.M., M.A.

7

Introduction

Rob A. P. Tielman, Manuel Carballo, and Aart C. Hendriks

The present and future course of Acquired Immune Deficiency Syndrome (AIDS) will depend largely on the dynamics of sexual transmission of the Human Immunodeficiency Virus (HIV) in the general population. One growing source of concern is the potential for transmission through bisexual contacts. Recent epidemiological data, particularly from Latin America and the Caribbean, document an alarming increase in HIV infection rates and AIDS cases among male bisexuals and their partners.

Continued high-risk behavior among male bisexuals in the AIDS era is believed to reflect their sexual isolation, low social visibility, and limited access to health promotion efforts. They are marginalized, and hence cut off from both mainstream heterosexual and targeted homosexual AIDS prevention campaigns.

Concerns for the bisexual route of transmission and the urgency of initiating health prevention efforts are compounded by an extensive gap in the knowledge of those who engage in sexual contacts with both female and male partners, the nature of their practices, and the context in which such contacts take place. Understanding bisexual behavior in the context of AIDS will depend largely on the extent to which the socio-cultural variations in its expression are made explicit.

This book is a first effort to assess current knowledge on bisexuality and to explore the relevance of bisexuality in the AIDS epidemic. Researchers in a wide variety of disciplines and representing nearly every region of the world generously collaborated to make an analysis of a specific aspect of the interrelationship between bisexuality and HIV/AIDS or to describe the (identified) patterns of bisexual behavior in their respective countries on the basis of currently available data and knowledge.

DEFINITIONS

Research on bisexuality poses a series of problems, many of which are related to operationalizing a definition of the behavior and identifying a population of "bisexuals." It is evident that socio-cultural differences in sexual practices and the formation of sexual identities are enormous and must be taken into consideration in our understanding of bisexuality.

A working definition was agreed upon: bisexual behavior as the involvement in sexual activity with both male and female partners over a certain period of time. In the epidemiological context of AIDS, it is male bisexuality that is of primary concern; yet female bisexuality may also have significance for the understanding of sexual cultures as a whole and the spread of HIV. A more precise definition of sexual activity and the retrospective time period referred to in the above definition will have to be determined in every factual research context.

It should be noticed that behavior is the key unit of analysis. Therefore the scope of interest should not be confined to the bisexual as a personality type or social category, bisexual behavior being much more common than its identification as such. Nevertheless, the development of a sexual identity and such labels as "homosexual," "bisexual," and "heterosexual" are central to our understanding of behavior.

PRELIMINARY FINDINGS AND CONSIDERATIONS

It is evident that existing knowledge of bisexuality is limited. Only a few studies, either of a qualitative or quantitative nature, have been conducted. While some studies on related topics, such as on homosexuality in certain population groups or sexual behavior in prison and in other segregated settings, touch upon patterns of bisexuality, the latter remains largely unexplored in social and behavioral science research. This is even true for societies or subcultures where bisexual practices either have become institutionalized or reflect accepted norms, though the actors are almost never referred to as "bisexuals."

As is the case in research, bisexual practices have rarely been exclusively targeted in HIV/AIDS prevention campaigns. Although the risks of HIV infection through certain bisexual practices ("high-risk be-havior") have been acknowledged, public health authorities have yet to address the problem. Lack of knowledge may be one of the major reasons for the failure of an accurate response.

Strong evidence suggests that male bisexuality is, and may increas-ingly become, an important factor in HIV transmission in several re-gions. From the existing data we learn that

1. while HIV prevalence data indicate that HIV seropositivity*
among bisexual men is, in general, lower than among homo-sexual men, it is higher than among heterosexual men;

2. men who have sex with men and women tend to engage in
high-risk behavior and, as a result, place themselves and their partners at risk of HIV. For example, studies have shown that bisexual men who have anal sex with men tend to have anal sex with women as well.

Bisexuality, much as exclusive homosexuality or heterosexuality, is a heterogeneous social phenomenon. Bisexual behavior in any par-ticular setting may involve a diversity of actors interacting over differ-ent time periods and for different objectives. Their lifestyles and sexual practices may vary in accordance. Despite this, a number of fundamen-tal patterns of bisexuality is reported to occur across societies.

Five "global" patterns of bisexual behavior that would enable cross-cultural comparisons are identified: the same- and opposite-gender sex-ual contacts of

a. youth;

b. men in an ongoing relationship with women (in some cultures
"married men");

c. men involved in male prostitution;

d. situational bisexual behavior; and

e. self-identified bisexuals.

Each of the above patterns entails specific concerns relative to HIV/AIDS. For example:

---

*The presence of antibodies in the blood following exposure to the AIDS virus (Ed.)

1. In many cultures, in anal sex young men tend to be more receptive, while older men more insertive.

2. The taboo on (homo)sexuality in many societies hinders sexual communication and therefore facilitates unsafe sex. This is particularly true in the case of "closeted" married men who do not disclose their same-sex contacts to their female partners.

3. A higher incidence of same-sex practices tends to take place in segregated institutions such as prisons and the military than in the general population. The repressive conditions usually associated with such institutions place individuals at higher risks of HIV infection. Group rapes, for example, are known to be frequent in many prisons, just as the nonavailability of condoms encourages unsafe sex practices among detained men.

Much of the risk behavior that bisexual men are involved in reflects their limited risk awareness or their tendency to deny same-gender sexual contacts. For example:

1. Bisexual men with unsafe sexual practices have been found to continue blood donations, whereas gay-identified men tend to refrain from doing so.

2. They are also less likely to ask to be tested for HIV antibodies at non-anonymous testing sites.

3. Among bisexual men who inject drugs, needle sharing may be perceived as high-risk behavior while safer sexual practices are not.

Many prefer not to disclose their same-and opposite-gender contacts out of fear of social (sometimes criminal) stigma. It is obvious that this hinders appropriate and effective HIV/AIDS prevention activities. Conversely, bisexual men who adopt sexual identities that reflect their sexual practices are more likely to respond to HIV/AIDS prevention campaigns.

1. In particular, those who actively participate in gay subcultures are more accessible to targeted prevention efforts.

2. Studies among youth with the same-gender contacts also indicate that those who identify as homosexuals are more accessible than those who identify as heterosexuals.

Finally, the distribution and expression of bisexual practices are found to be different across communities and social classes. For example, hidden bisexual practices are believed to be more common in traditional social orders encouraging "homophobic" attitudes than in those allowing for the expression of pluriform sexual lifestyles. In addition, expressions of sexual practices are more rigid in rural as opposed to urban areas, and more rigid among lower-class men compared to middle- or upper-class men.

RESEARCH QUESTIONS

It is important to generate knowledge of bisexual behavior in its different socio-cultural contexts and to measure to what extent patterns of bisexual behaviors in different cultures can be compared. This would enable a clearer understanding of the nature of high-risk behaviors and facilitate appropriate health interventions, notably HIV/AIDS prevention efforts.

A number of fundamental research questions emerges. These questions include:

a. How is high-risk behavior negotiated in interpersonal male-male and male-female relationships?

b. What relationship exists between bisexual high-risk behavior and the individual and/or social construction of sexual identities?

c. How is bisexual high-risk behavior embedded in socio-cultural norms and rules?

d. How can knowledge about bisexual behavior be transformed into effective AIDS prevention strategies for those involved in sexual contacts with both males and females?

THE SCOPE OF THE RESEARCH

To enable cross-cultural comparative studies, it is important that specific categories of bisexuality are the subject of research in different cultural settings. These studies should include cultures representing a diversity of regions in the world. Subject to local practices, and considering research feasibility that varies between regions, research should look at the following patterns of bisexuality:

a. adolescent males involved in bisexual behavior, particularly in the context of sexual experimentation;

b. men in ongoing heterosexual relationships involved in bisexual behavior that is usually undisclosed to the spouse;

c. gay and/or bisexual-identified bisexual men;

d. male prostitutes involved in bisexual behavior, both at work and in personal relationships;

e. the convergence of bisexual practices and substance use;

f. situational bisexual contacts as they occur in schools, detention centers, military barracks, and other segregated institutions ("institutional situational bisexuality"), as well as anonymous encounters such as while traveling, partying, etc. ("incidental situational bisexuality");

g. female and/or male partners of bisexual men;

h. age-group identified same-sex contacts, usually between obviously older and younger male partners;

i. transvestism, transgenderism, and transsexualism; and

j. females involved in bisexual behavior and their partners.

Specific issues that need to be addressed in research on bisexuality are:

a. sexual orientation and identity;

b. past, current, and "ideal" sexuality;

c. social class;

d. age, class, and ethnic-specific patterns of bisexuality;

e. active and passive sex roles;

f. unprotected anal sex with both male and female partners, as well as vaginal sex with female partners;

g. practices of condom use;

h. sexual techniques;

i. changes in sexual practices and identities over time;

j. stable relationships versus promiscuity;

k. simultaneous, concurrent, and serial bisexual behavior;

l. open versus closeted bisexual behavior;

m. cultural and ritualistic aspects of same-sex contacts;

n. social networks in which bisexual practices take place;

o. settings in which bisexual practices take place;

p. the development of social norms among persons engaged in bisexual behavior;

q. substance use;

r. practices of needle sharing;

s. sex tourism; and

t. HIV status.

To support the implementation of health interventions, specific attention should be given to the contents and evaluation of HIV/AIDS prevention strategies, and the way these strategies address and portray bisexual men, as well as HIV antibody testing as it applies to bisexuality.

RESEARCH STRATEGIES

To be able to enlarge our knowledge of bisexuality and its potential impact on the spread of HIV, diverse existing research strategies have to be adopted and combined in an international collaborative study of bisexual behavior. It is evident that only in the limited ccntext of certain Western urban centers can we speak of a self-identified bisexual lifestyle, a delineated community of bisexuals or of representative associations and institutions. For the majority of those who engage in bisexual behavior, no such clear social identity, support group, or localization exists.

Innovative research strategies are thus needed for studying an amorphous and, in many societies, secretive and discrete population group. The strategies should include:

a. On-site research that targets where high-risk sexual behavior takes place. Such sexual meeting points include bars, bathhouses, parks, and "street beats." Other sites include those frequented by self-injecting drug users and prostitutes.

b. Equally important is research on centers providing health care, family planning, STD and HIV antibody testing, and counseling services for those engaged in same and/or opposite-gender sex contacts.

c. The experiences and knowledge of key informants should be tapped. They include health educators and those integrated into bisexual networks.

d. Another source of considerable data are the AIDS information hotlines.

e. Institutions representing interests of bisexuals or those acting, whether openly or discreetly, as contact points in partner selections.

f. Conducting surveys of readers of and advertisements in specialized magazines, specifically erotic/sex magazines.

g. Addressing female partners of behaviorally bisexual men (e.g., in clinics or possible organizations).

h. Considering the data on subsamples of bisexuals derived from large-scale surveys, especially those conducted by WHO/GPA/ SBR* on Homosexual Males, Sexual Behavior, and Drug Injectors.

THE ELABORATION OF RESEARCH ON BISEXUALITY AND HIV/AIDS

The following recommendations are of crucial importance to enable cross-cultural research on bisexuality and HIV/AIDS.

1. Research should be conducted in a number of phases: a preliminary phase consists of an inventory of the current state of knowledge at both the global and the regional levels (this book is the first inventory of this kind), followed by exploratory quali-

*Socio-Behavioral Research

tative research on the crucial patterns of bisexuality (an international research project has been established to initiate and coordinate such a study); and finally, more structured qualitative and quantitative studies should be carried out on different population groups known to be engaged in high-risk bisexual practices.

2. Cross-cultural comparisons have to be assured through topic standardization rather than the identical wording of questions in the research instruments. Flexibility is recommended in the development of core instruments and research strategies. To obtain comparable findings, at least 20 interviews (consisting of a comparable core and optional modules) should be conducted among members of the same, or similar, target groups from different cultures.

3. Because of the difficulties seen in identifying respondents and accessing local networks, it is advisable that research be conducted by "insiders" addressing trusted representatives in the local setting.

4. Psycho-social research should be conducted independently of HIV prevalence studies on bisexuality. The collection of seroprevalence data poses numerous problems of feasibility, reliability, and ethical concerns and may jeopardize participation in a larger study. Thus, HIV testing should remain optional to those research sites that can justify that ethical considerations have been taken, including guarantees for confidentiality, informed consent, and the provision of counseling services.

5. Researchers conducting research on bisexuality, and in particular on people involved in bisexual behavior, must be bound by a statement of principles elaborated on the general WHO ethical codes for researchers.

STATEMENT OF PRINCIPLES FOR RESEARCHERS ON BISEXUALITY AND HIV/AIDS

It is already universally acknowledged that scientists conducting research are bound by scientific and ethical guidelines. To that end, codes of conduct have been developed on various occasions by different professional associations and organizations such as the World Health Organization. Besides these more general rules, specific guidelines may be considered necessary when research is conducted in sensitive areas or may lead to encroachment upon fundamental rights.

Given the stigmatization and discrimination, whether social or legal, directed toward individuals and groups adopting other than a heterosexual lifestyle, it is important that basic ethical principles operate, and are seen to operate, in any research on bisexuality.

Researchers who will participate in collaborative studies on this issue should subscribe to the following statement of principles and consider the points developed below in all stages of research.

1. The legal status of persons who engage in bisexual practices and who may consequently be at risk of HIV, should be protected. Respect for the enjoyment of human rights and fundamental freedoms should be guaranteed, independent of HIV status or sexual lifestyle.

2. It is the Human Immunodeficiency Virus (HIV), not individuals or population groups, that must be combated.

3. Discrimination against bisexuals undermines the development of relationships of trust with health care workers, health authorities, and AIDS researchers. In turn, such conditions weaken the fight against AIDS. As in the study of other subjects, a relationship of trust should be developed and maintained between respondents and researchers.

4. Counseling and other support should be given to those involved in bisexual practices and the bisexual community as a whole to prevent the spread of HIV, and adequate care should be guaranteed to those already infected.

5. Researchers should be fully aware of the implications of their findings (and the manner in which these are presented) on the social and legal status of those under study.

6. Research on bisexual behavior can only be conducted on the basis of voluntary participation and informed consent by respondents. Data should be securely stored and confidentiality has to be guaranteed. Researchers shall not pass individually identifiable data to any third person or use such data for any other end unless they have obtained the explicit, voluntarily given permission of those under study.

Part 1

Cross-Cultural Patterns of Bisexuality

1

A Taxonomy of Global Behavior

Michael W. Ross

Research into bisexuality has been done from a number of perspectives. However, the great majority of the work has been based on Western societies and has been psychological in orientation: that is, it has concentrated on motivations and personality variables in the individual, rather than on bisexuality as a social phenomenon. On the other hand, anthropological and historical analyses have examined bisexual behavior in cultural and temporal contexts and have paid greater attention to bisexual expression as influenced by socio-cultural considerations.

THEORETICAL APPROACHES

There are a number of extensive theoretical reviews of bisexuality (Hansen and Evans 1985; Klein, Sepekoff, and Wolf 1985; Morrow 1989; Paul 1985; Zinik 1985) that address the psychological issues in Western societies in some depth. However, all of these criticize the behavioral definition of bisexuality based on the bipolar continuum of Kinsey, Pomeroy, and Martin (1948). The so-called Kinsey Scale makes the assumption that because there is a scale with sexual partner preferences on it ranging from exclusively homosexual to exclusively heterosexual, there must be a bisexual entity (particularly as more people are behaviorally bisexual than are exclusively homosexual). A second problem with the Kinsey continuum is that being bipolar, it implies that the amount of homosexual behavior is a reciprocal of heterosexual behavior. This taxonomic approach has been criticized on the grounds that it only takes account of genital activity, and not affectional preferences. Unfortunately, the assumption that affectional preferences are central to sexual activity is itself culturally and temporally biased toward Western societies in the late nineteenth and twentieth centuries and is thus of limited use in examining global patterns of bisexuality.

Western research has attributed a number of etiologies to bisexual behavior: these include concepts that bisexual people are conflicted about whether they are heterosexual or homosexual, have retarded sexual development and have not yet developed to the point of making a choice between heterosexuality or homosexuality, or that they are using the self-definition as a defense against admitting to being homosexual. More positive perspectives see the bisexual person as being more flexible (Zinik 1985). However, as Morrow (1989) points out, human sexual orientation is not fixed, and thus assumptions of an immutable bisexual "identity" should not be made. Ross (1987) has argued that it is probably more cross-culturally appropriate to see people who have partners of both sexes as those who do not see partner gender as *relevant* to sexual encounters, thus de-emphasizing personality and psychodynamic explanations in favor of cultural and situational considerations. Similarly, Gagnon (1977) argues that it is important to examine the scripts that make sex with both genders possible. Cross-culturally, bisexual behavior will probably follow a number of scripts.

This discussion does not take any position as to whether homosexuality and bisexuality are essential or constructed conditions. It is based on the premises that there are degrees of interest in same and opposite sex partners and that individuals have the potential for erotic response to both. Freud (1905, 1961) held that sexual instinct existed independent of sexual object and that humans were born with innate biological potential. Ross, Rogers, and McCulloch (1978) suggested that individuals are socialized out of such polymorphous perversity and that the form of expression of their sexuality is culturally determined to a large extent.

CROSS-CULTURAL TAXONOMIC APPROACHES

Eight major patterns of bisexuality can be distinguished worldwide. These appear to be based on two major factors: first, the degree of stigmatization of homosexual behavior; and second, the degree of specialization of a homosexual role and opportunities for expressing such a role. The eight patterns proposed are discussed in turn.

Defense Bisexuality

In societies where a homosexual role is stigmatized, men may engage in bisexual behavior to (*a*) hide their homosexual activities; (*b*) use heterosexual activity as a base from which to explore homosexual activity; and (*c*) use bisexual behavior as a stage in the "coming out" process that is more acceptable personally and socially. Ross (1983) has described defense bisexuality as occuring in countries in which a homosexual orientation is stigmatized and leading to a greater number of marriages in homosexually active men. He found that more men who defined themselves as homosexual were likely to have been married or betrothed in more anti-homosexual Western countries. Similarly, Humphreys (1970) has found that many men who have homosexual encounters in public places and who are married display anti-homosexual and deeply conservative attitudes, including those toward homosexuality, and may be strongly religious. Ross (1978) found that men who identified as homosexual and who were married expected a strongly anti-homosexual response socially and personally, significantly more than those who had married but separated, who in turn expressed a significantly more negative societal reaction than homosexual men who had never married. He suggests that this putative societal reaction may be one explantation of defensive bisexuality.

Latin Bisexuality

Frequently in societies that are based on Mediterranean cultures, the homosexual role is conceptualized as taking the receptive (or feminine) role in sex. The individual who plays the insertive role is not conceptualized as homosexual and not stigmatized, provided he also engages in heterosexual sex (Carrier 1985; Parker 1989). The conceptualization of such behavior may also be dependent on age, with bisexual behavior that involves taking a receptive role more acceptable or less labeled in younger partners or where there is an age difference between the partners.

Ritual Bisexuality

In some societies homosexual contact has a ritual role in which older males will have homosexual contact with younger men as part of initiation rites. This contact may occur over a number of years, as in the Sambia of Papua-New Guinea (Herdt 1981). In this situation, the younger males act as fellators of older males in order to obtain the masculinizing effect of ingested semen. However, when they graduate to adulthood, they are in turn fellated. The practice apparently does not continue after marriage, when heterosexual relations commence.

In a similar situation, there may be homosexual behavior between a younger (usually adolescent) partner and a "mentor," where the mentor may also be married. Such behavior has been described among the Siwans of North Africa (Ford and Beach 1952) and in classical Greece (Dover 1978).

Married Bisexuality

Where marriage is regarded as a natural state and as part of family obligations, remaining unmarried is not an option for those who can afford it. In such circumstances, homosexual activity may take place anonymously away from the family living area in particular public locales. Examples of this pattern occur in India (Devi 1977). Kumar and Ross (1990) have noted that in India the majority of men engaging in homosexual contact had also had sex with women within the past few months and had a primary heterosexual partnership. This pattern is different from defense sexuality since there is virtually no alternative to marriage or life within an extended family, and marriage is seen not so much as a sexual institution but as a social one.

Secondary Homosexuality

Secondary homosexual activity may occur for reasons of lack of alternative outlets (as in single-sex institutions) or for financial reasons (as in the sex industry). Examples may include prisons (Wooden and Parker 1982), schools or military organizations, adolescent experimentation, and "hustling." In such cases there is often no homosexual (or bisexual) self-identification. In prisons, there may also be a component of expressing domination in insertive homosexual behavior: however, as this usually occurs within a setting that lacks heterosexual outlets, it is subsumed under the category of secondary homosexuality.

A second category of secondary homosexuality is described by Humphreys (1970) in men who may have sex in public toilets or parks with other men. Such contacts are usually anonymous and without verbal communication, and Humphreys describes them as being a sexual outlet "less lonely than masturbation." Given that, as Kinsey, Pomeroy, and Martin (1948) found, there are major class differences in the acceptability of masturbation, with those in the lower socio-economic strata seeing autoerotic activities as unacceptable or deviant, such behavior may be secondary to lack of acceptability of other outlets including autoerotic ones.

Equal Interest in Male and Female Partners

This pattern may occur in both Western and non-Western contexts. In developed nations, this is sometimes referred to as "true" bisexuality since the gender of the partner is not a particularly salient aspect of partner choice. In developing nations in which there may not be stronger strictures against homosexual activity as compared with heterosexual activity, or where there may be no concept of homosexual/heterosexual roles, the gender of the partner may also be less important than interpersonal or situational variables (Ross 1987). The category of equal interest comes closest to the "polymorphous-perverse" pattern postulated by Freud. In this category, availability of sex and situational factors may be stronger determinants than any sexual "self-identity": indeed, the self-identity may simply be "sexual."

Experimental Bisexuality

Adolescent experimentation may not always be secondary to lack of heterosexual contacts since it may occur despite available alternatives. Thus such experimentation is more like the pattern of equal interest in male and female partners. So-called inadvertent bisexuality that may occur under circumstances of inebriation or other disinhibitions can probably be described as experimental. The major characteristic of experimental bisexuality is that it may occur only once or twice in a lifetime and is usually not associated with a homosexual or bisexual identity.

Technical Bisexuality

Technical bisexuality may occur in the case of sex with prostitutes or other individuals who may present themselves as women or who may have had some form of gender reassignment. Nanda (1985) describes the Hijra of India, men who dress and act as women while being recognized as transsexuals. There are equivalents in a range of other cultures (Wikan 1977). While technically sex with transvestites or transsexuals may be considered to be bisexual in view of the sex of the individual, particularly where they are recognized as being a "third sex," it is usually not considered as "homosexual."

CONCLUSION

This chapter has attempted to provide a taxonomy of global patterns of bisexual behavior to help in the delineation and description of the phenomenon. It is based on the assumption that bisexual behavior is embedded within a social and cultural context that will provide different opportunities and different rewards and punishments for such behavior, and above all invest it with different meanings that will influence its form and frequency. Its usefulness as a tool for investigating the risks of HIV transmission and the modification of high-risk behaviors for sexual transmission of pathogens remains to be demonstrated. However, this taxonomy may also have some utility in the investigation of the effects of societal stigma, role, or identities that may underlie the expression of bisexual behavior.

2

Male Bisexuality and AIDS in the United States

Lynda S. Doll, John Peterson, J. Raul Magaña, and Joe M. Carrier

Until recently, data on homosexual and bisexual men have been aggregated in most AIDS-related research. The increasing number of AIDS cases attributed to heterosexual transmission (Centers for Disease Control [CDC] 1989) as well as preliminary data suggesting that some bisexual men continue to engage in high-risk sexual behavior and to donate blood (Doll et al. 1990a; Peterson 1989; Doll and HIV Donor Study Group 1990b) has prompted concerns that homosexual and bisexual men may represent distinct populations, each requiring targeted research and intervention.

Within the United States, very little is known about the population of bisexual men and their partners. Estimates of the size of the population are still largely derived from the Kinsey Reports of white men published in 1948. Furthermore, there is very little recent descriptive research on patterns of bisexual behavior in nonclinical populations, and comparison across the few available studies is difficult because of ambiguities in defining bisexuality (Klein, Sepekoff, and Wolf 1985).

To assist in the development of research and health interventions we present an overview of patterns of male bisexuality in the United States. We include, when available, recent data on AIDS-related risks in the various subgroups of bisexual men and discuss implications for accessing these groups. Because of distinct cultural influences on these patterns and because available data suggest that the AIDS-related risk may be highest among minority men (CDC 1986), special emphasis is placed on behaviorally bisexual black and Latino men, that is, men who report having sex with both men and women but who may self-identify as homosexual, bisexual, or heterosexual.

Since research focusing on bisexual men has lagged behind research on homosexual men, the data we present are often preliminary and not necessarily representative of the various subgroups of bisexual men. Generalizations from these data should be made cautiously. We have also drawn heavily from descriptive data from the authors' current research as well as presentations made at a workshop on bisexuality and AIDS sponsored by CDC in October 1989. We acknowledge the important contribution made by the participants of that conference, in particular John Gagnon.

IDENTIFYING BISEXUAL MEN

Self-reported measures of sexual identity have been used extensively to identify bisexual men (Coleman 1987). However, studies examining the relationship between sexual identity and sexual behavior suggest that a single measure of self-reported sexual identity may be inadequate and that multiple measures may be necessary to identify bisexual men. Data collected in a 1982 survey of approximately 7,000 *Playboy* readers showed that while 1 in 8 (13 percent) of those responding reported engaging in sex with both men and women, only 1 in 32 (3 percent) self-identified as bisexual (Lever 1989). Similarly, data collected in a recent study of HIV-seropositive male blood donors showed that among 129 men who reported having had sex with both men and women since 1978, 30 percent self-identified as homosexual, 34 percent as bisexual, and 36 percent as heterosexual. Behaviorally bisexual white men were more likely to identify as homosexual, whereas black and Latino men were more likely to identify as bisexual and heterosexual, respectively (Doll et al. 1990c).

BEHAVIORAL PATTERNS OF BISEXUALITY

The population of bisexually behaving men in the United States is diverse and includes persons engaging in a broad range of behaviors and patterns of interaction. These patterns vary by racial/ethnic background and social class. Furthermore, because bisexual behavior may be situationally defined, these patterns may change over the lifetime of individuals. To identify subgroups of bisexual men who could potentially be targeted for interventions, we have adopted a model suggested by John Gagnon (1989) that categorizes youth and adult bisexuals by their embeddedness within heterosexual or homosexual social networks. Such a model emphasizes behavioral patterns rather than motivations for engaging in behavior, and provides a potential context for developing intervention strategies.

BISEXUAL YOUTH

Bisexual adolescents and youth who are embedded within heterosexual social networks are often isolated and unaware of other homosexually behaving youth. As adults they usually assimilate into the mainstream heterosexual world and may or may not continue sexual contacts with both men and women. Because of the covert nature of this group of adolescents, few data are available on their risk behaviors or patterns of interaction.

A smaller, but more accessible, group consists of individuals who attend support groups for homosexually behaving youth in urban locations (Gerstel, Feraios, and Herdt 1989). The majority of these youth has engaged in sexual activities with both men and women during adolescence (Herdt 1989) with their sexual identity emerging as a part of the "coming out" process. Gay-identified youth in these groups tend to be only marginally involved in the heterosexual teen world and, as adults, may identify with urban homosexual networks. The extent to which youth self-identify as bisexual and the patterns of interaction among those who do are unclear. However, the existence of socially cohesive groups for these adolescents provides an opportunity for targeted risk-reduction education and the establishment of social norms regarding the importance of safe-sex practices.

AIDS-related data specifically on bisexual youth are limited. By February 1990, CDC had received reports of 161 homosexually behaving male adolescents ages thirteen through nineteen with AIDS. Eighty-one percent of these adolescents reported engaging in sexual activity exclusively with men, and 19 percent reported sexual activity with both men and women since 1978 (CDC 1990). Preliminary data on a sample of 63 primarily black and Latino male adolescents recruited from a New York City community agency serving gay youth are reported by Rotheram-Borus and Koopman (1989). Although only 8 percent of these youth reported bisexual activity in the three months before the interview, nearly 60 percent reported ever having had female sex partners. Though participants reported moderately high AIDS knowledge as well as beliefs endorsing AIDS prevention, the mean number of male sex partners during the three-month period was four with only 14 percent consistently using condoms. Data gathered at three- and six-month intervals after a multi-session intervention for these youth showed fewer youth engaging in a high-risk pattern of multiple sex partners, frequent sexual intercourse, and infrequent condom use (Rotheram-Borus et al. 1989).

ADULT BISEXUALS WITHIN HETEROSEXUAL SOCIAL NETWORKS

Bisexual men identifying with or embedded within heterosexual social networks may be divided into at least three subgroups: (1) men who are in primary relationships with female partners; (2) men who have sex with female partners but who are not in primary relationships; and (3) men who live in all-male institutional settings such as prisons. Although these men may vary in their motivations for sexual contacts with both men and women, and the extent to which they disclose these activities to their female partners, they generally lack the social cohesiveness of men embedded within homosexual social networks. Furthermore, to the extent that their male sexual partners are outside homosexual networks, they may also lack access to AIDS risk-reduction information targeted for gay men.

Except for limited data on sexual behavior in prisons, quantitative data describing the sexual behavior and social interactions of behaviorally bisexual men embedded in heterosexual networks are not available. Summarizing data on male prisoners, Gagnon and Simon (1977) estimated that between 30 percent and 45 percent have sex with other men while they are in prison. In a more recent study, Wooden and Parker (1982) found that 65 percent of a random sample of 200 male prisoners in a medium-security prison housing self-identified homosexual as well as other men reported having male sex partners during their current imprisonment. In total, 55 percent of prisoners who self-identified as heterosexual reported engaging in sex with men while in prison, including 42 of 52 black (81 percent), 17 of 31 Chicano (55 percent), and 27 of 71 white (38 percent) self-identified heterosexuals. The authors report that blacks and Chicanos were more likely than whites to play the dominant, inserter sexual role, suggesting that among these men, sex with men is condoned as long as dominance is maintained.

Sagarin (1976) reported limited data on postprison sexual identities of nine homosexually behaving ex-convicts, none of whom had engaged in sex with men prior to imprisonment. The five men who maintained a dominant, insertive sexual role in prison later reported resuming a heterosexual lifestyle. Perhaps because of the stigma in admitting same-sex behavior, the author was unable to locate men who had taken the passive, receptive role in prison and who subsequently resumed a heterosexual lifestyle. However, none of those located through homosexual social networks who had taken the passive, receptive sexual role in prison had resumed a heterosexual lifestyle.

Data from two studies suggest that female sex partners of bisexual men are frequently unaware of their partners' sexual contacts with men. In one study of 21 women who were married to bisexual men, only 3 of the 9 men who were aware of their sexual orientation before marriage had disclosed this information to their future wives. The wives of the remaining 18 men learned of their husbands' bisexuality a mean of sixteen years after they were married (Hays and Samuels 1989). Similarly, among 49 female partners of HIV-seropositive bisexual men enrolled in the California Partners' Study, 7 of 35 (21 percent) of the white, 4 of 5 (80 percent) of the black, and 7 of 9 (78 percent) of the Latina female partners were unaware of their partners' bisexuality at entry into the study (Padian 1989). A possible outcome of this failure to disclose is suggested in a study by Kegeles et al. (1990) of men seeking HIV testing at alternate test sites. These authors asked men under what hypothetical conditions they would be willing to be tested for HIV. Self-identified bisexual men were significantly less willing than homosexual men or heterosexual men and women to be tested for HIV if the names of HIV-seropositive persons were reported to public health officials. The authors suggest that fear of disclosure to their partners may motivate these bisexual men to avoid learning information crucial to both their health and that of their partners.

Data on AIDS-related risk specific to this population of behaviorally bisexual men embedded in heterosexual networks are also limited. By

February 1990, men who reported having had sex with both men and women since 1978 accounted for 19 percent of nonheterosexual persons with AIDS and 12 percent of all persons with AIDS in the United States. The extent to which these men were embedded within heterosexual or homosexual social networks before their diagnosis is unknown. However, 11 percent of women with AIDS who were infected through heterosexual contact reported sexual contact with a bisexual man. In addition, 2 percent of children with AIDS who were infected perinatally had mothers who reported sexual contact with bisexual men (CDC 1990).

Adult Bisexuals within Homosexual Social Networks

Bisexual men embedded largely within homosexual networks may remain marginal to the gay community as a result of political pressure from gay-identified peers regarding their bisexuality (Paul 1985). They may also be more likely to experience social pressure to engage in safe-sex practices, although social norms that have arisen within gay communities supporting safe sex may not extend to sexual contacts with women. Ekstrand (1989) found rates of unprotected anal sex with male partners declined by 72 percent between 1984 and 1988 among a group of 140 self-identified bisexual men living within a six kilometer square area in San Francisco heavily populated by gay-identified men and with the highest cumulative incidence of AIDS in that city in 1984. Ekstrand found that rates of unprotected vaginal sex declined just 58 percent during this same period among these men.

Adult Bisexuals within Homosexual or Heterosexual Social Networks

Men who have sex with men in exchange for money or drugs may be embedded within either homosexual or heterosexual social networks. Because of their frequent sexual contacts and drug use, they are at increased risk for acquisition and potential transmission of HIV infection. Among a group of 152 male street hustlers interviewed in a large city in the southeastern United States in 1988-1989, 71 percent self-identified as bisexual or heterosexual. Although the HIV-seropositivity rate was highest for self-identified homosexuals (40 percent), 31 percent and 15 percent, respectively, of those identifying as bisexual or heterosexual also tested HIV-seropositive (Elifson et al. 1989). Male hustlers who were behaviorally bisexual or who self-identified as bisexual were significantly more likely than nonbisexuals to use intravenous cocaine or heroin, to be homeless, and to have hustled in a number of large cities, perhaps on "hustler circuits." While these men had paid sex with men, they reported higher rates of recreational sex with women than with men (Boles, Sweat, and Elifson 1989).

There is no systematic research on the number or characteristics of men who identify with the small but active network of self-identified bisexuals throughout the United States. Furthermore, it is not clear how deeply this group of men identify with homosexual or heterosexual social networks. A directory provided by the East Coast Bisexual Network and the North American Bisexual Network lists approximately eighty support groups or centers available to bisexual men and women in urban locations. Newsletters such as *Bisexuality, Bay Area Bisexual Network Newsletter*, and *Boston Bisexual Men's Network (BBMN) News* have featured AIDS-related articles. In addition, a brochure prepared by the East Coast Bisexual Network emphasizes both individual safer sex practices and the cooperative efforts of bisexual and homosexual organizations to fight AIDS. While we have no data on AIDS-related risk in this subgroup of bisexual men, these organizations may have the opportunity to access and educate their members.

Black Bisexuals

Because the sexual behavior of minority men who engage in bisexual activities has rarely been studied, the frequency of these behaviors in black men is unknown. In fact, the extent of bisexual behavior among black Americans is largely derived from surveillance reports of nonwhite AIDS cases. Relative to the proportion of the total population, the incidence of AIDS among blacks is twice as high as among white homosexual and bisexual men (Bakeman et al. 1986; Bakeman et al. 1987; Selik, Castro, and Pappaioanou 1988). Of the homosexual or bisexual persons with AIDS, the percentage of persons reporting sex with both men and women since 1978 is 30 percent for blacks compared to 15 percent for whites (CDC 1990).

The high incidence of AIDS among black men attributed to bisexual behavior prompts the need for sexual data on these high-risk men. Currently, however, we are aware of only two studies that have reported data on the bisexual behavior of black men. Bell and Weinberg (1978) included data on the bisexual behavior of a small sample of black men (n = 111) in their study of homosexual males in San Francisco. While most of these men identified as homosexual, over 70 percent had experienced heterosexual contact at least once in their lifetime, including 20 percent in the year preceding the survey. In addition, these black participants had extensive same-sex experiences in which 90 percent had experienced receptive anal intercourse and over 75 percent had more than 250 partners in their lifetime. Recently, data have also been reported on the sexual behavior of a small sample (n = 47) of black bisexually identified men in the San Francisco Bay area (Peterson 1989; Peterson et al. 1989). While these men had a mean of over five male sex partners in the month prior to the interview, they reported a mean of fewer than two female sex partners during the same time period.

Many black men may have extensive sexual contact with both men and women without affecting their heterosexual identity. The proportion of bisexually active black men who identify as bisexual is influenced by cultural socialization and the lack of development of a black bisexual community. Typically, black Americans have disapproved of homosexual behavior, which has in turn inhibited public disclosure about such sexual activity. In one national survey, blacks were only slightly less approving of homosexuality than whites, although they tended to be much more tolerant of premarital sex (Klassen, Williams, and Levitt 1989). This disapproval of same-sex behavior, despite permissive attitudes toward opposite-sex behavior, may result in men having sex with both men and women without adopting a homosexual or bisexual identity. Others may protect themselves from the inference of bisexual identity, regardless of their bisexual activity, by exclusively engaging in only those same-sex activities that they consider to be masculine sexual roles (i.e., the inserter role in oral and anal sex) (Carrier 1985; Parker 1985; Wooden and Parker 1982).

Because the gay community in the United States is viewed by some blacks as being dominated by white men, in some communities there may also be an inherent tension between the development of ties to both the black and gay communities, respectively. Involvement in a gay community may be seen as a betrayal of the black community and thus may lead to severing of important friendship and family ties. This perceived choice between being black and being gay may lead to a rejection of the gay community in favor of a more bisexual lifestyle by some black men.

Black men who are behaviorally bisexual may also differ from homosexually identified men in their types of social networks. Black men who are bisexually active may have more frequent interpersonal relationships with heterosexual than homosexual peers. Also, many may have fewer homosexual peers in their social network than black homosexual men. These differences in social networks may influence how bisexual, as compared to homosexual, men recruit their potential sex partners. Thus, bisexual men may recruit partners among callboys, male hustlers, male prostitutes, transvestites, and anonymous men they meet in parks and adult bookstores. Black homosexually identified men may be more likely to select their sex partners from gay bars, bathhouses, gay clubs, and gay friends. These recruitment strategies may have important implications both for level of HIV-risk behaviors and for targeting AIDS risk-reduction programs.

LATINO BISEXUALS

The Latino population in the mainland United States is estimated to be close to 24 million, and while the majority are of Mexican (62 percent), Puerto Rican (12 percent), or Cuban (6 percent) origin (Strategy Research Corporation 1989), individuals may come from countries in Central and South America, Spain, and Portugal. Because of this diversity in country of origin, as well as differences in socioeconomic status and acculturation to mainstream Anglo culture (B. V. Marin and G. Marin 1990), considerable caution must be used when making generalizations about AIDS-related knowledge, attitudes, and behaviors within and between Latino populations.

Even greater caution must be used when making generalizations about male sexual behavior since most research to date has focused on only one segment of the Latino population: men of Mexican origin (Carrier 1985). A comparison of Anglo and Mexican male bisexuality, however, illustrates some important differences in behavioral patterns between the two populations, and it would not be unreasonable to expect that, unless highly acculturated, most Latino populations in the mainland United States should be closer to Mexican and Mexican-American patterns of homosexual and bisexual behaviors than to Anglo patterns.

One major difference in Mexican and Anglo homosexual behavioral patterns of particular relevance to the spread of HIV is that Mexican men generally have strongly developed preferences for anal intercourse over fellatio and usually have preferences for playing either the anal receptive or insertive sexual role (Carrier 1985). On the other hand, data suggest that most Anglo men do not have strongly developed preferences for playing one sexual role over the other and do not necessarily look upon anal intercourse as the preferred sexual technique in homosexual encounters (Bell and Weinberg 1978).

The dichotomization of sexual role preferences by Mexican men suggests that there may be at least two different male groups with homosexual contacts. By societal standards the one playing the anal receptive role is considered feminine and homosexual, and the one playing the masculine, inserter role is not. While homosexuality is traditionally viewed with disapproval within Latino populations (Singer et al. 1990), men who generally engage only in insertive anal intercourse are not stigmatized as "homosexual." Further, perhaps because of "machismo," the culturally defined hypermasculine model of manliness, there appears to be wide acceptance of the inevitability of multiple, casual sexual contacts from an early age including sexual contacts between men. The masculine self-image of a man is typically not threatened by his homosexual behavior as long as he engages in the appropriate sexual role and also has sex with women.

One important outcome of this dichotomization with respect to the spread of HIV is that a larger percentage of men of Mexican origin may be involved in bisexual behavior than Anglo men. This is reflected in recent AIDS case data showing that among the homosexual/bisexual cases reported to the CDC, 22 percent of the Latino, as compared to 15 percent of the Anglo cases, reported having sex with both men and women since 1978 (CDC 1990). Carrier (1985) estimates that as many as 30 percent of Mexican men between the ages of fifteen and twenty-five may engage in sex with both men and women.

Magaña and Carrier (1988) have examined the extent to which bisexual behaviors change when Mexican men move to the mainland United States. Preliminary analysis of interview and observational data from their study of Mexican and Mexican-American sexual behavior suggest that even though patterns of sexual behavior among immigrant Mexican men are somewhat modified by new and quite different socio-cultural factors, their homosexual behaviors in California continue mainly to be patterned on their prior sexual experiences in Mexico. Interviews of 52 immigrant male Mexican farm workers in southern California, for example, revealed that 23 percent had been involved in homosexual behavior.

However, Magaña and Carrier also suggest that as a result of the greater availability of female sex partners in the United States, due to dramatic changes in courtship practices in Latino communities where there is less regulation of female sexual behavior by families and societal norms than found in Mexico, fewer Latino males may be involved in bisexual behavior. At the same time, with the reduced family and community controls of sexual behavior and with the availability of organized gay communities in many urban locations, some Latino immigrants to the United States may choose to be exclusively homosexual.

While acculturation over time may reduce the extent of bisexual behavior in Latino men, the risk of HIV infection in this population continues to be high. The favored sexual practice with male partners is anal intercourse (Carrier 1985). Since many of these men do not consider themselves homosexual or bisexual, they represent a potentially difficult group to reach through educational intervention designed for Anglo gay men. Additionally, since the Latino population in the United States is made up of people of varying degrees of acculturation and scholastic attainment, effective intervention programs must allow for different outreach intervention strategies.

ACCESSING MALE BISEXUALS FOR RESEARCH AND INTERVENTIONS

The number of identifiable subgroups of bisexual men, as well as the distinct cultural influences on their behavior, suggests that multiple intervention strategies will be necessary to encourage behavior change in these populations. The model proposed by Gagnon also suggests that to intervene effectively with subgroups of bisexual men, it is necessary to take into account the relevant social networks and, in particular, the extent to which the individual or his partners identify with gay communities.

Men who themselves or whose partners are connected to gay communities may continue to be the most accessible for AIDS education efforts. However, because bisexual behavior is stigmatized within some gay communities, interventions may be needed to decrease this stigmatization and to support social norms for protecting both male and female partners. Increasing the visibility of organizations specifically designed for bisexuals may also provide an additional source of risk-reduction information for men who do not identify as homosexual.

Adolescent or adult bisexual men who are primarily embedded within heterosexual social networks may be less aware of their risk for HIV than men who are involved in homosexual social networks because of the lack of AIDS information sources and the opportunity to discuss information within their primarily heterosexual social networks. These men may also be much harder to reach for AIDS interventions because they are not involved in socially cohesive groups with social norms encouraging safe-sex practices.

Schwartz (1989) suggests that among these men, individuals whose same-sex contacts are (1) infrequent, (2) not recent, (3) not emotionally salient, (4) not central to their identity, or (5) not perceived as actual sex with a man, may be particularly hard to access. Strategies aimed at reaching these men through the workplace or family (Marin, Marin, and Juarez 1990) are essential. Disseminating risk-reduction messages close to sites of sexual activity such as bathhouses, restrooms, or rest stops may also be effective, since interventions in close proximity to the sexual activity may be more likely to be attended to and may also reinforce any social norms for safe sex operating at that site. To reach black and Latino men, community interventions must be developed that include their group-specific values, norms, and expectations (Peterson and Marin 1988; Marin 1991; B. V. Marin and G. Marin 1990). Also, these interventions must consider antihomosexual attitudes that may prevent many black and Latino bisexuals from either receiving prevention information or from accepting it if received.

Although male hustlers may be physically accessible for research and interventions, preliminary data suggest that drug use and possibly transiency must be taken into account in interventions aimed at this population. Furthermore, interventions need to address both paid sex with male partners and recreational sex with female and male partners.

The extent to which male bisexuals may be accessed through female partners is unknown. Data we have reviewed would suggest that few women are aware of their partners' behavior; hence, female partners may not form a cohesive, targetable group. Cultural taboos against both sexual communication between men and women and the perceived control of male sexuality by women may also discourage women from introducing safer sex practices into relationships where disclosure has occurred. On the other hand, to the extent that the needs for emotional intimacy and family closeness of bisexual men are met through relationships with women, female partners may have some power over sexual decision making. Most importantly however, because male bisexuals may separate their sexual lives into two discrete worlds, it is crucial that educators develop interventions targeted separately for sexual activities with male and female partners.

TARGETING RESEARCH ON BISEXUALITY

Our review has highlighted the need for additional research to understand both bisexual behavior and identity in general, and, more specifically, the relationship between bisexuality and HIV infection. To understand adequately why bisexual men may continue to put both themselves and their female and male partners at risk for HIV, it is essential to understand first the patterns of bisexual behavior within the United States. With this foundation, we will be able to develop effective AIDS risk-reduction programs. Critical issues related to male bisexuality and AIDS that should be addressed include (1) the incidence of sexual behaviors with male and female partners; (2) the extent of, and factors related to, disclosure of same-sex sexual behaviors or sexual identity to female partners; (3) social and sexual networks of bisexuals, including the extent of their identification with ethnic or homosexual communities or organizations specific to bisexuals; (4) factors related to behavior change and perception of HIV-related risk; (5) cultural or ethnic differences in bisexual behavior; and (6) the relationship between sexual identity and sexual behaviors. Furthermore, to implement these data on male bisexuality within minority communities, additional research is needed to assist in the design and implementation of culturally appropriate AIDS prevention strategies.

CONCLUSION

Scientific understanding of the epidemiology of HIV infection in the United States would be incomplete without the cooperation of homosexual men who have generously given their time and divulged intimate aspects of their lives for scientific research. The data we have presented support the need to pursue additional behavioral research on male bisexuality and AIDS. To develop a research partnership with bisexual men, scientists must understand the individual and cultural constraints that influence their behaviors and avoid blaming individuals for transmission of HIV infection from homosexual to heterosexual populations.

3

Bisexuality in Mexico: Current Perspectives

María de Lourdes García García, José Valdespino, José Izazola, Manuel Palacios, and Jaime Sepúlveda

INTRODUCTION

Since the appearance of the first AIDS case, the urgency to control what has become a rising epidemic among the Mexican population has given impetus to a great number of investigations. In view of the widespread practice of bisexual sex in this country and the consequent possible HIV transmission through high-risk techniques, research on this facet of the problem has become a top-priority target for analysts.

Practical research on bisexuality has been from its inception a highly complex field, not only from the medical and epidemiological viewpoint, but even more so from the perspective of sociological, political, psychological, and ethical factors that, in the composite, provide important clues to Mexican sexuality and lifestyles.

Initial steps in the research were geared to analyzing the relationships or correlation between bisexual practices and the growing AIDS epidemic. On the heels of this introductory phase socioepidemiological studies followed that analyzed knowledge and attitudes toward AIDS and their relation to sexual practices and HIV prevalence. The most recent approach has been qualitative studies that explored in depth the varied circumstances surrounding and characterizing bisexual practices and their influence on the lifestyles and standards of the practitioners.

41

Results of the epidemiological analyses were insufficient to reveal accurately the complexities of the problem. The frequency and incidence of bisexual contact among the population were impossible to ascertain. Qualitative studies have offered valuable sociological and psychological information about some groups with bisexual practices, but others remain to be investigated. However, despite this gap in the exploratory data, investigators have established certain facts that have indisputably pointed to bisexual activity in specific segments of the society.

Now the campaign for the prevention of AIDS is seeking profound and accurate information relative to the activities in question. It is mandatory to assign priorities to the study of behavioral practice different from the socially accepted "norms," and to direct the public toward awareness and prevention with regard to this epidemic.

FACTORS PERTINENT TO BISEXUALITY IN MEXICO

The role of sex partners, man and woman, relative to their sexual conduct together, and·to the influence each has over the other in establishing their behavioral code is of prime importance to this survey. To begin with, the Mexican attitude toward sexual relations is excessively lenient toward the male, granting him virtually uncensored behavior in whatever relationship he chooses. This is the foundation on which is fabricated the fabled Latin American "machismo." This term implies a kind of free-swinging bravery, fortitude, courage, and daring and, of course, dominance. Machismo is much admired by most Mexicans including the women. Tacit approval and even encouragement is given to the pubescent boy's initiation into sex. The permissiveness of his elders, and peer pressure exerted by his own age group lead frequently to promiscuity and later on to a polygamous standard for sexual relationships.

In contrast, women are placed primarily in two categories. First, the good woman embodies man's lofty ideals of the "faithful wife, devoted mother, and accomplished homemaker." She must be a virgin before marriage, and she is virginal after marriage, untouchable by anyone other than her husband. At the other extreme is the bad woman, identified by gradations of unworthy behavior. She is unattached, pleasure-giving and pleasure-seeking, is permissive and undemanding of her sex partner, and shows no signs of modesty, patience, and prudence, those most revered attributes of the good woman. And finally, at the bottom of scale, there is the prostitute, the ultimate "bad" girl.

One result of this stereotyping is the young man's dilemma when he reaches the age of initiation into sexual activity and discovers that no "good" girl or woman suitable for him is available. Either he must pay a prostitute or pursue his sexual life with males—men of his family perhaps, a cousin or brother, or more likely with boys who are friends and neighbors. He can enter into a homosexual relationship, assigning himself the role of penetrator, thus keeping his "macho" image intact. His guard is up against acquiring any identification as being gay. He takes the position that his maleness will not be jeopardized so long as he plays the active role. He may even convince himself that his masculinity is reinforced by his homosexual insertion and then certainly reaffirmed by his casual sexual exploits with women.

On the other hand, there is also the receptive role played by the homosexual, whose identity is seen as effeminate, and who is relegated to the status of the typical Mexican woman in relation to her husband or lover. In any case, the effeminate role when played by the male suffers taboos and stigma from the social, cultural, and religious standards of behavior. But the careful delineation between the homosexual who only engages in insertive practices and the one who plays only the receptive role is becoming more tenuous and therefore less inhibiting. Men who engage in both practices used to be known as "international." With the advancement of the gay movement has come increasingly liberal acceptance of variant sexual behavior. Thus, the adoption of exclusively active or passive roles is increasingly less frequent (as further discussed below).

But entrenched social forces still militate against overt adoption of alternative lifestyles. An additional factor to be examined in Mexico is the prevalent low level of sex education. Investigators see this as one of the imponderables in a prudish, tradition-bound, male-oriented society. Most Mexicans have little accurate knowledge of their sexuality—the transmission of diseases through sexual contact, the scientific approach to family planning, the use of condoms, to mention but a few of the many areas of ignorance that are pervasive regarding sex in this country. These matters are often equated with taboos and myths, and, to complicate the problem further, it is culturally in bad taste to discuss openly the vagaries of intimate behavior.

Another aspect of the problem can be found in the custom of group socializing in exclusively male company. It begins when the boy or adolescent attaches to a peer group or club that offers various attractions such as sports, parties, games, and, above all, companionship. This type of recreation is most often encountered among adolescents before marriage. After marriage, however, many men continue their all-male socializing as though they were still single and free to enjoy the exclusive company of their *cuates* or buddies.

Finally, family acceptance is eminently important to the Mexican and he adapts his behavior to the standards set by his upbringing. Homosexuality in this context is viewed as suspicious and shameful; the homosexual, then, is careful always to appear before his family as a heterosexual. He will "prove" his "normalcy" by having girl friends and eventually taking a wife.

THE BLUEPRINT OF BISEXUALITY IN MEXICO

Mexican bisexuals must be observed on a wide spectrum where a very wide variety of sexual practices takes place. The following information covers some of the more frequent types of male bisexual activity.

The Gay Man

The gay community in Mexico has recently begun to surface or, as they state it, "come out of the closet." Gays are organizing with the mutual goals of achieving public and legal acceptance, and they are proclaiming their rights through private and public channels. The typical member of this group is young, a student or comparatively new in his career, and he is apt to be a professional and/or an intellectual. He chooses to live in the big city where he can escape rejection and stigma from small-town society in general and from his family in particular. The Mexican gay, more often than homosexuals in other countries, will establish relationships with women, some of them lasting. Less frequently, he will resort to female prostitutes for the sake of his image or will have occasional sex with women in the business world or in some branch of education. At the other end of the spectrum is the member of the gay community who participates with loud voice in public demonstrations, protest movements, publicity campaigns and, not least, patronizes recreational clubs devoted exclusively to gay clients.

Not infrequently however, he has not accomplished a complete self-identification and will try to maintain a "normal" presence among heterosexual family associates, and to achieve this he will have heterosexual relationships. In his sexual practices with men, he finds that the distinction between active and passive roles is becoming less clear. He often tries sexual techniques that may result in HIV transmission—such practices as rectal douches or fisting. In his sexual encounters with women, anal intercourse and fisting are also frequent. The use of the condom is not widespread, and on the occasions when it is used, it is with a male partner. Members of gay communities have acquired considerable information on the transmission, treatment, research progress, and prevention of AIDS. Surveys on knowledge, attitude, and practices have shown that, nevertheless, there is still a wide gap between awareness and prevention among these groups.

The Married Homosexual or Bisexual Man

In contrast with the gay man who is obviously identified as such, there is the man, homosexual or bisexual, who refuses to admit or indicate his sexual preference before the world. In other words he takes pains to remain "in the closet." From the beginning of his sex life he has taken both male and female partners, the episodes with males having been occasional and usually anonymous. After he is married he will continue to have furtive sexual affairs with men. He will hide, however, and for fear of disclosure will seek his partners among nameless prostitutes or street waifs. At other times his homosexual activity will take place in the company of male friends who are carousing and drinking together. In this ambiance his sexual encounters will be entirely penetrative, rather like an exercise, thus reminding himself and his companions that in truth he is not really gay.

Street Children and Male Prostitutes

City streets are home to many children, almost all boys, who have been abandoned or have run away. They earn a little money at marginal jobs—car washing, vending candies or chewing gum—and a fair number of them subsist on what they can glean from petty thievery. An alarming percentage of these youngsters sniff glue or use some other mind-altering inhalants. They conduct their activities in groups of three or more, and, as protection from the police, attach to adolescent gangs whose survival depends on shady pursuits beyond the law. They bond together in a kind of fraternity and initiate sexual activity as often with females as with males. In pairs and sometimes alone they prostitute themselves for clients who are usually married men. These gang youths often are blurred in their sex preferences, and some will adopt the effeminate role and then be called by their associates the *loquitas pobres,* poor little crazy-girls.

"Macho" Prostitutes

The term *chichifo* refers to a type of young man from the lowest economic level, who earns his living as a prostitute serving male clients, usually from medium- or high-economic strata. His main characteristic is his "macho" image. He exaggerates his masculinity, tends to be violent and defiant, and reaffirms his maleness often by flaunting his relations with female partners who are also prostitutes.

Circumstantial Prostitution

Numbers of heterosexual men in the low-income bracket work in gay establishments as bath attendants, masseurs, porters, janitors, gym instructors, and for additional income will prostitute for the men who habituate such places. Most of these workers are married and do not look upon their prostitution as homosexual per se. They see it as simply an easy way to add a bit more money to the family's maintenance fund.

Also involved in male prostitution are indigenous natives from Indian groups in the provinces who have migrated to urban centers seeking job opportunities. They accept any kind of work that usually pays no more than the minimum wage—basic construction work, street vending, street cleaning, and anything else they can get that they can physically handle. In the city they soon learn that prostitution is another economic source and they will solicit homosexual clients, usually men from the upper classes who travel to low-class districts for anonymous sex with males. Still another segment significant in AIDS transmission is made up of Mexicans who have entered the United States legally or illegally, for better wages than they can hope to find in Mexico. They discover that in addition to the dollars they earn as migratory workers, they can amass even more to send home to their families if they engage in homosexual prostitution from time to time.

Youth Gangs

Belonging to a "gang" is for many adolescents from slum-dwelling families an escape from their environment, which is fraught with hostility, violence, and grinding poverty. Although heterosexual by preference, they often engage in homosexual practices as part of their "rite of passage," that process they must go through in order to become a member of the gangs' "inner circle." They learn the codes, willingly submit to orders, and do anything, including homosexual sex, to ingratiate themselves with the bosses.

Indigenous Bisexuals

Among indigenous tribes, particularly those of Veracruz, State of Mexico, and Puebla, homosexual practice is regarded as a form of sexual initiation. In other groups, in the southern part of the country, the married man adopts an adolescent boy who is proud to have been chosen for the honor of being used as the older man's lover. In addition to serving sex on demand to his master, the boy will also help the master's wife around the house and with the children. When the boy reaches adulthood, his circumstances will follow those of his former master. He will marry and procreate and very likely engage a young boy to do for him what he used to do for his former sponsor. He has come full circle.

Situational Bisexuals

In certain environments, homosexuality is practiced by heterosexual men for the simple reason that women are not available. This situation exists in prisons, barracks, military training, on board merchant or war ships at sea, or on petroleum rigs offshore.

Self-Identified Bisexuals

The bisexual is rarely identified as such in Mexican society, even though he is found on all levels, from high to low, of the socio-economic structure. Individuals attempting self-classification as bisexual find it not only futile but also unacceptable to the public. They are rejected as much by the gay community as by the heterosexual segments of society. The revealed bisexual probably loses his heterosexual as well as his homosexual partner. He must try, therefore, to satisfy his bisexuality by having sex only with others of the same persuasion. In the conduct of bisexuality, the man will have partners of both sexes, and probably will establish a stable relationship with both. Depending on his partners' willingness to accept his bisexual activity, he may have stable arrangements with both a woman and man at the same time. Occasionally a case is found in which the bisexual shares his household with both partners. Recently, bisexual groups have organized among urbanites for mutual support and understanding, and for workshops where sexual problems can be aired and analyzed informally and in a nurturing environment. These groups are relatively few. Not many bisexuals dare to affiliate with other bisexuals for fear of disclosure.

FREQUENCY OF BISEXUAL PRACTICE IN MEXICO

We do not know accurately the extent of bisexual practices in Mexico. Some investigators, such as Carrier, estimate that around 30 percent of males between the ages of fifteen and twenty-five have at some time or other engaged in this practice. Other studies, however, indicate lower percentages.

The Ministry of Health made a survey of the male population in 1987–1988 to establish a picture of prevalent sexual practices. Five hundred subjects from the age of 15 to 60 years and residing in any one of six big cities were interviewed. Two percent had homosexual sex and 0.4 percent admitted bisexual practices. In previous and subsequent surveys, in the period between 1985–1989, 5,040 Mexican men, self-identified homosexual, were polled. Sixty-seven percent maintained heterosexual relationships in addition to homosexual ones. This group resides in towns of less than 100,000 inhabitants. The other group that lived in metropolitan areas including Mexico City revealed that 56 percent had relations with both sexes.

From these statistics, it is surmised that in Mexico the percentage of men who have sex with men is similar to that of other countries; for instance, in the United States the Kinsey report indicated that 4 percent of the male population were exclusively homosexual in their relationships. In Mexico, on the other hand, the frequency of sex relations with women by avowed homosexuals is higher percentage-wise than in the United States. We know still less about the frequency of bisexual practices among married men or among self-identified bisexuals. But there are hints that suggest that bisexuality is perhaps a widespread sexual practice in Mexico, not necessarily linked to bisexual self-identification.

FIGURE 1
Trends of Transmission Categories in AIDS Cases
Mexico, 1983–1991

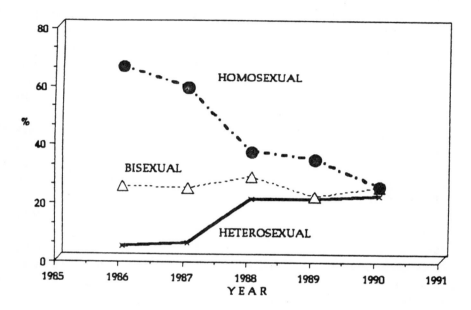

THE RELATION OF BISEXUAL PRACTICES
TO THE HIV/AIDS EPIDEMIC IN MEXICO

The first 17 AIDS cases registered in Mexico during 1983 occurred in homosexual and bisexual men of the high economic level who lived in Mexico City and who had traveled internationally. At present, the total number of AIDS cases is 6,510 as of March 1991. Cases have been seen among children and adults throughout the country.

As is the case in other countries, the majority of cases are associated with sexual transmission, which represents 81 percent of adult cases. Of this 81 percent, 40 percent are homosexual men, 24 percent bisexual men, and 17 percent heterosexuals. Analysis of the trends of homosexual, bisexual, and heterosexual transmission shows important differences. Homosexual transmission represented 65 percent of total AIDS cases up to 1986; during the first three months of 1990 this percentage decreased to 25 percent. Cases associated with bisexual transmission have remained stable. Heterosexual transmission has had a rapid growth, from an original figure of 4 percent in 1986 to 20 percent (fig. 1).

This increase among heterosexuals is seen as the product of two factors: first, the transmission of infection by men whose practice is bisexual; and, second, transmission of contaminated blood transfusions by heterosexual recipients who later infect their partners. Since 1986 control over the blood supply has been widespread, and now it appears that bisexual practices have become the most significant factors in heterosexual transmission.

Two additional facts point to the importance bisexual practices are having on HIV transmission. One of these is the number of newborns with AIDS whose fathers are active bisexuals—the current figure with regard to this factor is 19 percent. Second, an important proportion of cases classified as heterosexual may really be bisexual men.

Therefore, if the trend of transmission categories in male AIDS cases is analyzed, it can be seen that a decrease has been noted among cases associated with homosexual practices, while an increase among cases due to heterosexual, blood, and perinatal transmission has occurred. Bisexual cases have remained stable. However, if a proportion of heterosexuals is really bisexual, an increase also exists in this category.

QUANTITATIVE STUDIES OF BISEXUAL PRACTICES AMONG MEN

Since 1985 the Mexican Health Ministry has undertaken a program of quantitative studies of homosexual and bisexual men. The investigation has probed areas of seroepidemiology and factors inherent in the attitudes, knowledge, and sexual practices related to AIDS. These studies have led to an epidemiological portrait of HIV transmission among selected groups in the main cities of the country. Investigators are now sorting out findings to evolve ways and means for educational intervention programs.

Sociodemographical Characteristics of Groups Under Study

The methodology for recruiting persons suitable for study has shown that the majority are members of the group known in street language as "gays of cabarets." These subjects are by definition homosexuals and

bisexuals who frequent night spots catering specifically to the gay patron—establishments such as bars, discotheques, and night clubs. During
the period from 1985 to 1990 more than 5,000 men in this classification were under study in 18 cities. Of course the groups in the probe,
i.e., the gays of cabarets, obviously represented only a narrow segment
of the homosexual and bisexual population. The study excluded, for
example, those men who refuse to admit their bisexual-homosexual
practices through fear of stigma or of losing employment, prestige, or
family acceptance. It also excluded men with homosexual and bisexual
practices who live in rural areas. It behooves one, therefore, to take
into account that a subgroup, rather than the entire group, was the
focus of this scrutiny. Taking this limitation into consideration, one
sees some very interesting conclusions that came to light after the investigation was documented. It was found that the frequency of bisexual
practices was slightly different from city to city according to the size
of population. The highest percentages were found in small communities
where 67 percent of men with homosexual practices also have sex with
women. In metropolitan areas such as Mexico City this same category
showed 56 percent of 1,657 men who adopted a bisexual pattern.

In comparing bisexual subjects with those whose sex practices are
exclusively homosexual, it was shown that although the age of the two
groups was more or less equal, the level of education and socio-economic
status was definitely unequal. They were considerably lower among the
bisexuals (table 1). It was also observed that bisexual men in little towns
tend more to establish stable relationships with women (30 percent versus
16 percent) and to have children (28 percent versus 15 percent) than
those of the same sexual classification in larger cities.

Certainly this finding indicates that the social and economic level
of the individual significantly influences the quality and quantity of his
sex life. It appears that bisexual activity among homosexual men is
more frequent in groups where homosexuality per se is ostracized and
where "machismo" in its more flamboyant expression is looked upon
as desirable. In this type of environment, the confirmed homosexual
must hide behind heterosexual relationships. In contrast, the big city
environment does not exert the same inhibiting pressures and, therefore,
bisexuality is not caused so much by the need of the individual for
acceptance.

TABLE 1
Sociodemographic Variables Among
Mexican Homosexual and Bisexual Men

	Bisexual Men 925 (56%)	Homosexual Men 732 (44%)	P Value*
Age	28.5 (sd 8.4)	28.8 (sd. 7.4)	NS
< Elementary School	10%	7%	< .05
Rural and Indus-try Workers	4%	2%	NS

*T Test, chi-square test. NS: Not significant

Source: General Directorate of Epidemiology, Ministry of Health, Mexico

Sexual Practices of the Bisexual Men

In analyzing bisexual practices from the standpoint of age of initiating sex with males, it is found that among homosexuals and bisexuals it is more or less the same age, thirteen years, for initiating sex with males. Another finding of interest indicated that insertive intercourse, i.e., "active," and receptive or "passive" anal intercourse were both practiced by the same individual. Seventy-seven percent of bisexuals engaged in "passive" anal intercourse and 95 percent in "active" intercourse. In their sex with men, 72 percent of bisexuals practiced fellatio; 32 percent cunnilingus; 17 percent fisting; and 10 percent rectal douches. These percentages were nearly the same for exclusive homosexuals. Wide differences, however, were noted between homosexuals and bisexuals in the number of sex partners they have in a given time. On the average, bisexuals have fewer lifetime male partners than homosexuals—110 versus 170 (table 2).

In analyzing the bisexuals' relations with women, the poll showed that the majority waited until they were twenty years of age or older to have sex with women. After this starting age, the average number of women partners during the previous six months period was two. In this group, vaginal intercourse is frequent (97 percent); anal intercourse much less (37 percent). The frequencies of fellatio, cunnilingus, and fisting with women by the bisexual was 46 percent, 20 percent, and 19 percent, respectively (table 3).

TABLE 2
Sexual Practices by Mexican Homosexual and Bisexual Men

Practice	Homosexual Men (n = 732)	Bisexual Men (n = 925)
Receptive Anal Coitus	95%	77%
Insertive Anal Coitus	88%	95%
Fellatio	89%	72%
Cunnilingus	36%	32%
Fisting	24%	17%
Rectal Douches	12%	10%
STDs	53%	53%
No. of Male Partners Median (Range)	170 (1–5,000)	120 (1–7,000)
HIV Prevalence	35%	28%

STD(s): Previous Sexually Transmitted Disease(s)

Source: General Directorate of Epidemiology, Ministry of Health, Mexico

---

TABLE 3
Sexual Practices by Mexican Bisexual Men with Women

Practice	Frequency (n = 925)
Vaginal Coitus	97%
Anal Coitus	37%
Fellatio	46%
Cunnilingus	20%
Fisting	19%
Stable Relationship with Women	16%
Had Children	15%
No. of Female Partners Median (Range)	2 (1–5,000)

Source: General Directorate of Epidemiology, Ministry of Health, Mexico

TABLE 4
Sexual Practices and HIV Prevalence Among
Bisexual Men According to Gender of Partners*

	Males Partners (n = 673)	Male and Female Partners (n = 325)	Female Partners (n = 115)
HIV Prevalence	31%	23%	21%
Receptive Coitus	89%	75%	46%
Insertive Coitus	94%	94%	70%
Rectal Douches	14%	8%	2%
Previous STD	57%	51%	51%
No. of Lifetime Partners Median (Range)	25 (1–7,000)	15 (1–5,000)	3 (1–3,000)
Anal Coitus with Women	38%	43%	19%
Stable Relationship with Women	6%	21%	47%
Had Children	5%	19%	33%
No. of Lifetime Female Partners Median (Range)	3 (1–400)	3 (1–400)	12 (1–5,000)

*During previous six months

Source: Seroepidemiological Survey, General Directorate of Epidemiology, Ministry of Health, Mexico

When sexual practices among bisexual men during the six months prior to the investigation were analyzed according to the gender of their partners, it was found that practices that carried risk for HIV infection were more frequent among those who had related only with men, intermediate among those who had related with men and women, and lower among those who had related only with women. Those who had engaged only in heterosexual practices tended, more frequently than the other two groups, to be married, to have children, and to have

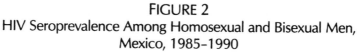

FIGURE 2
HIV Seroprevalence Among Homosexual and Bisexual Men,
Mexico, 1985-1990

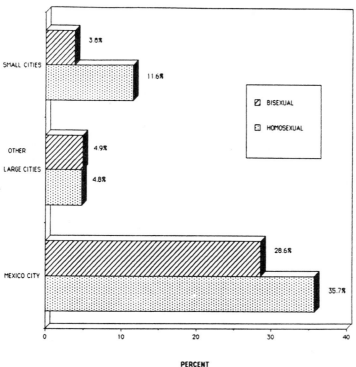

more female partners. Compared with the other two groups, they practiced anal coitus with their female sexual partners less frequently (table 4).

Prevalence of HIV Infection and Risk Factors

The prevalence of HIV positive antibodies in the bisexual men under study was highest in Mexico City—28 percent. The least number of positive tests were in small communities, 5 percent, and middle-size cities, 4 percent. In all cases combined, HIV prevalence was lower in men with bisexual practices than in men having sex only with men (fig. 2).

The prevalence of HIV infection is rising in various cities under study. In 1985 homosexual and bisexual men living in Mexico City showed 5 percent infected with HIV; in 1986, 23 percent; in 1987, 33 percent; and in 1988, 38 percent. A similar rise has been noted in other cities:

56   Cross-Cultural Patterns of Bisexuality

TABLE 5
HIV Risk Factors for Bisexual Men

Risk Factor	% with the Characteristic		OR	CI	P Value*
	Seropositive (n = 268	Seronegative (n = 657)			
Anal Receptive Coitus	88	74	2.66	1.73–4.11	<.01
Rectal Douches	17	8	2.46	1.55–3.9	<.01
STD	61	50	1.6	1.18–2.16	<.05
>10 Male Partners	77	63	1.94	1.37–2.77	<.05

OR: Odds Ratio; CI: Confidence Interval, 95%
*Chi-square test
STD(s): Previous Sexually Transmitted Disease(s)

Source: General Directorate of Epidemiology, Ministry of Health, Mexico

for example, the HIV infection rate in Acapulco, the famed tourist mecca, rose from 0 percent in 1986 to 10 percent in 1988. In Tijuana, on the northern border, the figures were 10 percent in 1986 and 15 percent in 1988.

Analysis of the frequency of infection among bisexual men varies according to the gender of the partner during the last six months of this investigation. The largest percentage was shown in those subjects who had related sexually only with other men (32 percent). Among men whose relationships had been exclusively with women the percentage was lower, 21 percent, and in the intermediate group whose subjects had sex with both genders, the percentage was 24 percent. Studies have also been performed among other groups of men with bisexual practices. HIV prevalence among male prostitutes has ranged between 6 percent in small cities and 16 percent in Mexico City. Among street children living in Mexico City seroprevalence was found to be 4 percent.

Considering sexual practices in relation to the risk involved, there is a similarity noticed between men who are exclusively homosexual and those who are bisexual regarding risk factors associated with HIV infection. The practices in question for both groups are receptive anal intercourse, rectal douches, previous sexually transmitted disease and having 10 or more partners. For men engaging in these practices, there is a two or three times greater possibility for infection with HIV than for men who don't engage in these sexual practices (table 5).

Knowledge and Attitudes Toward AIDS and
Their Interrelation with the Adoption of Preventive Measures

The search for knowledge, attitudes, and practices relating to AIDS undertaken by the Ministry of Health has included, besides the polling of homosexuals and bisexuals, extensive examination of other groups including prostitutes, students, health personnel, and, last but not least, the general public.

Analysts have found that bisexual men, allied as they are in their forms of sexual practice to strictly homosexual men, possess quite extensive information with regard to the etiology of AIDS, the modes of its transmission, and the measures for its prevention. The level of knowledge about AIDS among this group is higher than that in other groups. In spite of this, however, the influence of myths and misinformation is relatively high. One out of every five bisexuals interviewed believed that daily contact was sufficient for infection, and one out of three thought that HIV was transmitted by mosquito bites. The attitude toward groups whose practices were in the high-risk category revealed a good level of acceptance. An appropriate level of risk perception was also found.

Differences in information and attitudes were not apparent between those whose practices were exclusively homosexual and those who were bisexual. However, it was also revealed that as many homosexuals as bisexuals continued with high-risk practices even though the participants were aware of the dangers. Of those questioned 66 percent stated that they were afraid of infection. However, 42 percent declared that in any case they would have sex with a recent acquaintance. Dissociation between knowledge and attitudes and sexual practices is more evident when the use of condoms and other preventive measures are analyzed. In the practices researched, it was noted that more than 95 percent of bisexual men were familiar with the condom but only 58 percent had used one during the previous months, and only 24 percent always practiced "safe sex."

FINAL CONSIDERATIONS

The life-and-death urgency to control AIDS has brought out in the open themes that once were considered taboo for social conversation, for public advertising, for the ears of children, and for popular reading. But now discussions at any level and by means of any media are mandatory. The most recent facet of this problem poses the question about the frequency among the population of bisexual activity—that is, how pervasive is it in Mexican society? There is evidence that bisexual practices in the Mexican fabric are more widespread than in other countries, the reason possibly residing in cultural and psychological phenomena. In Mexico, bisexual practice is not specifically identified with sexual preference on the part of the practitioner, and its underlying implications are not what they seem at first glance.

Estimates on the extent of bisexual practice raise the question of what pressures or sociological forces are at work in modifying it. In this traditional society, homosexuality and bisexuality are branded as stigmas, shameful aberrations prohibited by the standards of decency. Could this condemnation that is so unyielding have something significant to do with the characteristics of bisexual behavior? How do social and family pressures exert psychological and behavioral influence on the individual's decision to adopt a bisexual identity? These questions among many others are still to be examined and analyzed in depth. At this stage of investigation it appears that the practice of bisexuality is a complex phenomenon that interacts with multiple variables at both individual and social levels.

What effect has bisexual practice had on the spread of HIV infection and AIDS? What percentage of bisexuals have been infected, and what percentage of AIDS cases in general can be traced to bisexuality? The answers to these questions are still problematical, but there does seem to be a tendency to equate the rise of heterosexual AIDS cases with the prevalence of bisexual sex. And this fact or surmise raises another critical point: to what degree have women, the heterosexual partners, been infected by their bisexual male partners? An increase in HIV infections is presently being noted among heterosexuals. What role is the bisexual playing in this statistical picture?

We are now facing a serious challenge—how can bisexuals be reached by programs for the prevention of AIDS? Health educators must consider the masculine and feminine roles played by bisexuals, their non-self-identification, either as homosexuals or as bisexuals, and the dissociation between knowledge and attitudes toward AIDS, and adoption of preventive measures. The growing AIDS epidemic throughout the world demands an all-encompassing and profound campaign to understand it. This campaign must include as a priority studies of bisexuality and bisexual practices.

4

Bisexual Behavior and HIV Transmission in Latin America

Richard G. Parker and Oussama Tawil

Although bisexual behavior has been linked to HIV transmission in a number of different parts of the world, there is mounting evidence that it has played an especially important role in the emerging HIV/AIDS pandemic in Central and South America, in parts of the Caribbean, and among Latinos in the United States.

In all these areas, early attention focused on the spread of HIV principally through homosexual contacts, and bisexuality was initially treated as little more than a subgenre within the category of homosexual transmission. Early attempts to interpret the spread of HIV in terms of the three major patterns of transmission that have characterized the international AIDS pandemic (Piot et al. 1988) quickly ran into serious problems, however, when confronted by an increasingly complicated epidemiological reality. While HIV transmission in the region as a whole was initially classified as part of Piot et al.'s Pattern I, this was quickly revised in the Caribbean, where heterosexual transmission showed a sharp enough increase to warrant reclassification, along with the countries of Central and West Africa, as part of Pattern II. And although homosexual transmission has continued to play a central role in the spread of HIV in Central and South America, even there, by the end of the 1980s, increasing rates of heterosexual transmission have led to a reclassification of the region to the newly invented Pattern I/II (Chin and Mann 1990). Finally, even though the United States has continued to stand as the leading example of Pattern I transmission, it has become apparent that the spread of HIV among Latinos (and other ethnic groups within the broader U.S. population) may have more in common with HIV transmission in many Latin American societies than with the dominant pattern in the United States itself.

While there may be a number of other important factors involved as well, it seems clear that much of the confusion that has been involved in attempting to categorize and characterize HIV transmission in the Latin American world (broadly defined as including the Caribbean and Latinos in the United States) can be linked to the role that bisexual behavior has played in the spread of HIV infection (see Cortes et al. 1989), and to the difficulty with which bisexuality seems to be incorporated into the conceptual models that are used to interpret and understand HIV and AIDS not only in epidemiological but also in social and behavioral research (see Parker 1987). In both Mexico and Brazil, for example, throughout the AIDS epidemic, roughly 20 percent of the reported cases of AIDS have been classified as bisexual males (see García García et al. 1989; Rodrigues and Chequer 1989; Valdespino et al. 1989). In Brazil it has even been suggested that at least some cases currently classified as heterosexual transmission may in fact be behaviorally bisexual men who fail to report same-sex contacts (Castilho et al. 1989). Roughly 15 percent of the cases of AIDS reported to the Caribbean Epidemiology Center from throughout the Caribbean region have been classified as bisexual (Narain et al. 1989; Hospedales and Mahibir 1989), as have between 10 percent and 15 percent of the cases recorded in some Central American nations such as Honduras (Beach et al. 1989). Throughout the region, this relatively high frequency of HIV infection among bisexual men has also been linked, in turn, to a series of additional complications. In Brazil, for example, anal intercourse between bisexual males and their female sexual partners has been identified as an important factor in HIV transmission among women (Sion et al. 1989), while roughly 20 percent of the cases of pediatric AIDS thus far recorded have been in children with bisexual fathers (Bergamashi et al. 1989), suggesting a rather different picture of vertical transmission than that found in other regions. In short, although other factors (such as IV drug use and, in particular, poorly controlled and tested blood supplies) have not been altogether absent in the spread of HIV in Latin America, it seems clear that bisexual behavior has played a major role in shaping the changing epidemiology of AIDS throughout the region (see Parker 1990b).

What is perhaps most striking here, however, is not simply the importance that bisexual behavior seems to have assumed in the epidemiology of HIV and AIDS in Latin America, but the extent to which this is in fact understandable in light of social and behavioral research on patterns of sexual behavior in the region. Long before the emergence of the HIV/AIDS pandemic, anthropologists and sociologists working in Latin America had pointed to a distinct construction of sexual interactions throughout the region in which occasional (or even relatively frequent) same-sex interactions need not necessarily call into question male gender identity. On the contrary, for a variety of complex reasons that may well differ slightly from one Latin American society to another, it would nonetheless appear that throughout the region an individual's role in same-sex contacts may actually be more important than his choice of sexual object. Carrying out what is perceived as the active role in both sexual intercourse as well as gender performance, even in cases of sex between men, need not undermine an individual's basic male identity, and the distinction between active and passive roles is in fact more important throughout the region than are the medical or scientific classifications of homosexuality, heterosexuality, and bisexuality. Perhaps most important, an individual's same-sex interactions do not necessarily inhibit or even influence his sexual interactions with members of the opposite sex (see, for example, Carrier 1971, 1976, 1985; Fry 1982, 1985; Fry and MacRae 1983; Lancaster 1988; Parker 1987, 1988, 1989, 1990a; Pinel 1989; Taylor 1985).

Given this understanding of Latin American sexual culture, and of the social construction of sexual interactions between men in much of the Latin American world, the role played by bisexual behavior in the spread of HIV comes as no surprise. On the contrary, long before epidemiologists had begun to rethink the classification of Latin America within their tripartite system, social and behavioral researchers had pointed to the importance of bisexuality and had suggested that current epidemiological categorizations would be inadequate in characterizing HIV transmission in Latin America and Latin North America (see Carrier 1988; Carrier and Magaña n.d.; Parker 1987, 1990b). Equally important, social researchers and health educators have pointed to the urgent need for a more sophisticated understanding of Latin sexual culture in order to develop more meaningful and culturally sensitive interventions for AIDS education among Latin American and Latino populations (see

Carballo-Diéguez 1989; de la Vega 1989, n.d.; Magaña et al. n.d.; Parker 1988).

In light of these considerations, it is clear that social and behavioral research on bisexual behavior and the social and cultural construction of bisexuality should be taken as a key priority within the Latin American region. Attention must focus, for example, on developing a fuller understanding of both the similarities and differences in the construction of bisexual behaviors throughout the region, and the social forces that may structure them. Rural and urban differences will no doubt be important throughout the region, as will differences in social scale, with more highly developed and diverse subcultures linked to same-sex interactions emerging in the urban areas of large-scale societies such as Argentina, Brazil, and Mexico than are found in smaller-scale, more predominantly rural societies. Similarly, specific variations or particularities in the social and cultural reality of different nations will clearly be important as well, as in the case of Costa Rica, where an unusually developed middle-class shapes same-sex interactions in ways that may contrast with the more class-stratified situation found in Brazil, Mexico, or Peru. Finally, the ways in which different societies are positioned within wider social and economic systems can have an important impact, as in the case of Puerto Rico, Haiti, or the Dominican Republic—all relatively smaller-scale societies in which the complexity of sexual subcultures and behavioral patterns may nonetheless approximate larger-scale contexts due to the impact of the world economy and tourist industry.

An understanding of the important particularities or differences that may be found in the construction of bisexual behaviors and realities throughout the Latin American world, however, should also be linked to an attempt to identify cross-national patterns that may ultimately serve as a focus for comparative research. While they are not the only patterns that may ultimately emerge as important in this area, nor are they necessarily limited to Latin American cultures, even a brief review of the existing literature is nonetheless sufficient to point to a number of specific patterns that might serve as a focus of research attention within the region. Bisexual behavior on the part of married men, both male and transvestite prostitution, adolescent sexual experimentation, the sexual behavior of street youth, and situational bisexuality in prisons and other institutional settings have all been identified in the existing research literature as important behavioral patterns in many parts of Latin America and the Caribbean, as well as among Latino populations in the United States. These aspects of bisexual behavior might conceivably offer important areas for comparative, cross-national research on bisexual behavior in relation to HIV transmission and AIDS.

Ultimately, then, the changing shape of HIV/AIDS epidemiology in Latin America should draw our attention to the role that social and behavioral research can play both in identifying and understanding the socially and culturally patterned behaviors involved in HIV transmission, as well as in providing a foundation for socially and culturally sensitive and meaningful health promotion and intervention strategies. If research on bisexuality generally should be taken as an urgent priority due to the serious lack of knowledge and understanding that we possess on what is often a particularly hidden or covert form of human behavior, then research on bisexuality in Latin America should be taken as an especially high priority precisely because of the salience that bisexual behavior has assumed for an understanding of the HIV/AIDS epidemic in this area. It offers us the opportunity of making a major contribution to the fight against AIDS through the development of comparative and collaborative research initiatives.

5

Bisexuality in the United Kingdom

Mary Boulton and Tony Coxon

INTRODUCTION

Until the AIDS epidemic focused attention on risk behaviors, the nature and extent of sexual behavior in Britain was of little interest to either medical or social researchers. Concern to understand the potential dynamics of the epidemic has since given rise to a number of studies of sexual behavior, but bisexuality still remains a neglected area of research. This in itself reflects the way bisexuality is viewed in Britain: it does not exist as a socially legitimate, or even socially recognized, way of life.

Despite a veneer of tolerance, attitudes toward homosexuality in the United Kingdom remain suspicious and hostile, as recent legislation makes very clear. Among the general (heterosexual) population, any same-sex contact is stigmatized and marks an individual as "homosexual," while within the homosexual community the homosexually active are also pressured to take a stand as exclusively "gay." Neither community recognizes the legitimacy of bisexuality. This has inhibited the development of a distinct bisexual community with the result that individuals outside London or Edinburgh who engage in bisexual behavior have no public reference group and little basis on which to form a clear social identity. They tend to remain as isolated individuals with limited contact with other bisexuals, invisible within the broader heterosexual and homosexual communities. Our knowledge of bisexuality in Britain is therefore largely opportunistic, coming from studies of sexual behavior in these two broad groups. Ethnographic research on bisexuality as such is only just beginning, and our understanding of the range of people and practices involved is still limited.

RESEARCH ON BISEXUALITY

Epidemiological Studies of Homosexual and Bisexual Men

The most systematic information on the extent of bisexual behavior in Britain comes from two large-scale community studies of homosexually active men: the Health Behaviour Research Project (Fitzpatrick et al. 1990) and Project SIGMA (Davies et al. 1990). These studies indicate that most homosexually active men have had sexual contact with women at some time in their lives, although the age at first contact with females suggests that much of this may be limited to the early years of sexual activity and the process of "coming out" as gay (table 1). A much smaller proportion of men continue to be actively bisexual: about 10 percent in a year and 5 percent in a month. These figures are very similar to those obtained in other surveys and are probably a good estimate of the incidence of bisexuality among homosexually active men in England and Wales. What is less clear is how far these figures indicate the existence of a distinct and stable population of bisexual men separate from the population of homosexual men. Bisexual men are much more likely to be, or have been, married (about 30 percent compared to less than 10 percent of homosexual men), and there is some evidence that they may be younger (Davies et al. 1990) or more middle class (Fitzpatrick et al. 1990). However, there may be few differences in attitudes and behavior among older bisexual and homosexual men.

    In terms of sexual identity, Fitzpatrick et al. (1989) found that about 9 percent of the homosexually active men thought of themselves as bisexual. Interestingly, the correspondence between sexual identity and sexual behavior was not good: a third of the men who thought of themselves as bisexual had not had sexual contact with a woman in the previous year, while almost half of those who had had a female partner in the previous year did not think of themselves as bisexual. Similarly, Davies et al. (1990) found that only a quarter of behaviorally bisexual men put themselves at points 2 to 4 on the Kinsey scale of feelings and attractions.

TABLE 1

Heterosexual Activity among Homosexually Active Men

	Fitzpatrick et al.	Davies et al.
% having female partner in lifetime	52	61
age at first sex with female—mean	18	18
—range	12–45	4–70
% having female partner in last year	10	12
number of female partners—mean	1	4
—range	1–7	1–200
% having female partner in last month	4	5

In terms of sexual behavior, there are few differences between bisexual and exclusively homosexual men in patterns of sexual behavior with men. Fitzpatrick et al. (1989) found similar rates of active (insertive) anal sex in the previous year (about 60 percent) and slightly lower rates of passive (receptive) anal sex among bisexual men (45 percent compared with 62 percent). Unprotected anal intercourse occurred more frequently with regular than with nonregular male partners. A third of the men never used a condom with regular partners (34 percent as the active partner, 31 percent as the passive partner), and a fifth never used condoms with other partners (16 percent as active, 16 percent as passive). Looking at behavior in the last month, Davies et al. also found only slightly lower rates of anal intercourse among bisexual men (25 percent compared with 30 percent for active anal sex; 22 percent compared with 28 percent for passive anal sex). Half the men never used a condom with regular partners, a fifth never used condoms with casual partners in active anal sex, and half never used condoms with casual partners in passive anal sex, though numbers here are very small.

Among the behaviorally bisexual, the mean number of female partners in the previous year was between 1 and 4. Fitzpatrick et al. found that almost all had had penetrative vaginal sex, 73 percent with regular female partners and 30 percent with other female partners. Of those who had vaginal sex, a third never used a condom with regular partners and over half never used a condom with other partners. Over half the men in Project SIGMA who had had vaginal intercourse with a woman in the previous month did not always use a condom. Anal intercourse was relatively rare among the men in this study (less than

10 percent had ever engaged in it), though more common among the men in the Health Behaviour Project. About a fifth of these men (16 percent) had had anal sex, usually with their regular female partner, and half never used a condom. These data suggest that while changes have occurred in high risk sex with male partners, high rates of unsafe sex persist with female partners, particularly nonregular partners.

While the scale of these studies means they are valuable in providing basic epidemiological data, there are limitations in their aims and methods with regard to understanding bisexuality in the United Kingdom. The samples are drawn largely from the population of self-identified gay men, the research focus is on sexual behavior with men, and even with large samples, the numbers of bisexual men recruited are small. Epidemiological studies such as these need to be supplemented by more qualitative studies of samples of men recruited specifically as bisexuals.

Descriptive Studies of Bisexual Men

A more descriptive account of bisexuality is provided by a small-scale exploratory study, still in progress, of men who had had both male and female partners at some time in the five years prior to interview (Boulton et al. 1989). Men were recruited from a number of different sources (clinics for sexually transmitted diseases, gay pubs and clubs, contact magazines, bisexual groups, and contacts of interviewees) to ensure that as wide a range as possible was included in the study. The aim was to explore the diversity of experience and behavior among these men who, in the context of this anthology, are grouped together as bisexual. The following discussion is based on the first 35 men interviewed.

Looking at the men's sexual history, six distinct patterns were identified. These reflect differences in the men's ages and social situations as well as in the numbers and types of partners they have had and the context in which they met. They also have implications for the men's sexual identity, both "private" and "public," and for the kinds of issues they face in managing their sexual relationships, particularly with women.

The first pattern ("transitional") was found among four of the younger men and reflects the process of "coming out" as gay: an initial period of exclusively or predominantly heterosexual activity is followed by a period of exclusively homosexual activity. These men now think of themselves as gay and intend to continue to have sexual contact exclusively with men, though some are unwilling to rule out the possibility of relationships with women again in the future. An example is Andrew, a thirty-year-old librarian, living with his male lover of three years. As an adolescent he had been attracted to other boys, which worried him, but at university he had found a girlfriend whom he lived with for several years. He had several subsequent girlfriends, one of whom was bisexual and who encouraged him to explore his own homosexual feelings. He joined a gay organization and has since had three regular and several casual male partners.

The second pattern ("unique") was found among five of the older men who had established a pattern of exclusively homosexual or hetero-sexual activity but then "deviated" from this established pattern on one or two occasions. In some cases, this was related to the disinhibiting effects of alcohol or drugs: for example, Allen, a thirty-four-year-old man who had been exclusively gay for 12 years got drunk at the office Christmas party and went to bed with one of the secretaries. In other cases, it was a physical expression of emotional involvement in one special friend. An example is Brian, a twenty-three-year-old laborer with a steady girlfriend, who had had a sexual relationship with his best male friend for several years. The friend had been killed in a motor accident, and Brian had never felt attracted to any other men.

In none of these cases did the "deviant" activity affect the men's sexual identity: all thought of themselves as gay or straight, in accordance with their predominant pattern of behavior. Perhaps for this reason, disclosure of the "deviant" activity was not seen as a problematic issue, though for some this meant ignoring it and for others, discussing it with their current partners.

The next four patterns reflect a more active level of bisexual behavior.

The third pattern ("serial") was one of alternating (but not over-lapping) periods of homosexual and heterosexual activity. Three men showed this pattern. They were younger and had had relatively few partners of either sex. The sexual identity they stated at interview reflected the sex of their current partners and may have changed with different phases of sexual activity. An example is Chris, a twenty-six-year-old telephone technician, currently with a regular male partner. In the pre-vious six years he had had four male and three female partners, with none of the sexual relationships lasting more than a few weeks. He had met his partners at school and then at university where he joined the campus bisexual group, which he continues to attend.

The majority of men in the sample showed a pattern of overlapping periods of homosexual and heterosexual activity: that is, the men had both male and female partners through most of their sexually active lives.

There are three variations on this theme (patterns four to six), reflecting the varying "communities" in which the men led most of their lives.

The fourth pattern ("concurrent: straight") was of men having long-term relationships with women but continuing to have male partners at the same time. These men thought of themselves as bisexual but maintained a "public" identity as heterosexual. All four of the married men in the sample were in this group, together with three other men who lived with their female partners. Most had a regular male partner; some had casual male partners as well. An example is Douglas, a forty-three-year-old business man, married with two children. He was no longer sexually active with his wife but in the last year had had over 60 male partners whom he met through contact magazines. His wife knew that he had had male partners in the past, but he had agreed not to do so after they married, and she was unaware of his current homosexual activity. The other married men were more open with their wives about their male partners, though the one who also had other female partners concealed this from his wife. For the unmarried but cohabiting men, disclosure of their male partners appeared more problematic, and only one was open about his current partners. This was Edgar, a twenty-six-year-old student living with his girlfriend of four years. During their relationship he had had three male partners, met through college or college friends, all of whom were known to her and grudgingly accepted.

In the fifth pattern ("concurrent: gay"), the men were active members of the gay community but regularly and frequently had relationships with women as well. There were 11 men in this group, roughly half of whom thought of themselves as gay and half as bisexual. An example is Freddie, a forty-four-year-old company director living with his male lover of 16 years. He had three other regular male partners and numerous casual male partners and had just ended a two-year affair with a thirty-five-year-old woman, an executive in his own company. Like other men in this group, he was openly gay and all his female partners knew about his homosexual activity from the beginning. Another example is George, a twenty-two-year-old student with a male lover and 20 other male partners in the last year, as well as two female partners, one of whom was a good friend from college whom he saw for several months, the other a "one night stand" after a party. He was active in the "gay scene," openly bisexual, and assumed that both his male and female partners knew and accepted this.

In the last and least common pattern ("concurrent: contact magazines"), three men had large numbers of both male and female partners over extended periods of time. Two thought of themselves as bisexual, one as "unrestrained" and all were involved in networks of other homosexually active men approached through contact magazines. An example is Henry, a sixty-year-old college lecturer, divorced but living with a woman of fifty-four. As a couple they used contact magazines to meet other couples for sex parties. However, unknown to her, he also used contact magazines to meet male partners. In the past year he had had 18 male and 24 female partners. A younger example is John, a twenty-three-year-old hotelier, who in the last year had had 3 regular and 4 casual female partners as well as 10 male partners. He met his girlfriends through work and parties and used contact magazines to meet other men for casual sex.

It is interesting to note that while there is no "bisexual scene" in the United Kingdom equivalent to the "gay scene," there are both "bisexual groups," which meet annually at a bisexual conference and contact magazines that cater to bisexuals among other groups. There appears to be little in common between them, however, with those attending bisexual groups being concerned more with sexual and personal identity and the option of having relationships with both men and women, and those using contact magazines being more concerned with meeting casual sexual partners.

BISEXUALITY AND HIV INFECTION

From the beginning of the epidemic in the United Kingdom, homosexual and bisexual men have constituted the largest group of AIDS cases. At the end of December 1990, 79 percent (3,234) of people with AIDS were homosexual or bisexual men, as were 65 percent (8,597) of people testing HIV antibody positive. Official figures published by the Public Health Laboratory Service do not distinguish between homosexual and bisexual men. Studies based on a variety of STD clinics, however, suggest that the prevalence of HIV seropositivity is lower among bisexual compared with homosexual men (table 2).

CONCLUDING REMARKS

What earlier research there is on bisexuality in Britain has either examined the Freudian notion of a protean bisexual identity or has con-

TABLE 2

Prevalence of HIV Antibody in Bisexual and Homsexual Men

	Bisexual %	Homosexual %
Welch et al. (1986) (criteria not specified)	5.1	17.9
Evans et al. (1989) ("frequently heterosexual" and "predominantly homosexual")	5	30
Collaborative study group (1989) ("sexual preference")	South East Thames	
—1986	6.0	17.4
—1987	9.5	16.2
	Other Regions	
—1986	4.0	6.8
—1987	.7	3.4
Project SIGMA (1990) (Sex of partners in last year)	5.6	9.9

centrated primarily on (heterosexually) married gay men. But sexual behavior and sexual identity are often markedly out of conjunction in the case of bisexual men: those behaviorally bisexual may avow or refuse the label, and those who accept the label may in fact behave in a different way. We cannot therefore rely on subjects' avowals to delineate bisexuality.

Since our focus is necessarily behavioral—HIV transmission can only occur via behavior, not identity—we have restricted attention to "those who have sex with men and women." What we now know, primarily from studies of men who have sex with men, is that the amount of male/female sexual contact among this group (almost all high risk, if not protected) is considerable: more men engage in it, and have more contact, than has been realized. But there are also distinct *patterns* of bisexuality, and we know little about the frequency of these types and less about patterns of change between the types. Yet each type has potentially different consequences for transmission in this important "bridge group" between the other two main sexual constituencies.

Manifestly, future research cannot afford to ignore this differentiation within bisexual behavior nor treat "bisexuality" as an unproblematic residual phenomenon. It poses problems of unique importance.

6

Bisexuality in the Netherlands: Some Data from Dutch Studies

Theo G. M. Sandfort

As in most other countries, in the Netherlands bisexuality has not been the subject of in-depth research. Only since bisexual behavior was seen as the major potential bridge between the gay population infected with HIV and the uninfected straight population, has it become a topic of interest for AIDS prevention policy makers.

The official figures about the prevalence of AIDS cases in the Netherlands give no clear picture of the importance the role of bisexual behavior in spreading the virus. As of January 1, 1991 there are 1,531 diagnosed AIDS cases in the Netherlands. In Europe, the Netherlands ranks seventh in the number of AIDS cases per capita: 106.5 per one million inhabitants. In comparison, the United States has 611.3 AIDS cases per million inhabitants. Of all the diagnosed cases in the Netherlands, 79.9 percent belong to the category of gay and bisexual men. Unfortunately, there is no subdivision between gay and bisexual cases. Additionally, with respect to women, no specifications are given about the ways in which they have become infected.

BISEXUALITY IN THE AIDS ERA

In the Netherlands no specific attempts have been made to reach bisexual persons to teach them about the prevention of HIV transmission (Moerkerk and Elbers, see chapter 14 of this volume). Items on bisexuality in relation to AIDS were included in the campaign directed at the general public, assuming that the message would also be understood by persons who have sex with men as well as women. Bisexual men have also been approached within the different activities directed to divergent target groups like homosexual men, male prostitutes, prison inmates, seamen, blood donors, and so on. Moerkerk and Elbers state that prevention directed at bisexuals should not be dependent upon whether they form a bridge between the gay groups and the population in general.

However, since policy makers are lacking the data and insights on the basis of which they can design their activities, the need for well-founded data became clear. These data go beyond the prevalence of bisexual behavior. Also important is an overview of the different forms in which bisexuality is practiced as well as insights into the ways the behavior is imbedded in sexual identities and regulated by cultural norms. Bisexuality has been set on the research agenda, as the AIDS threat did with several other forms of sexual expression as well.

BISEXUALITY RESEARCH

To the extent that data about bisexuality are available at this moment, they are generally to be found in surveys directed at much broader topics. Two kinds of data are available: data that are related to the way people experience themselves or label their sexual attraction, and data that refer to actual sexual behavior, whether or not it is labeled by the person as bisexual. If bisexuality is being studied in the form of behavior, one has to define an arbitrary time frame in which sexual contacts with persons of both sexes should have taken place, in order to classify the behavior as bisexual. It is clear that too long a period —e.g., lifetime behavior—renders the concept of bisexuality meaningless. Just for the sake of practicality, a period of five years has been chosen in this study.

Witte (1969) has been one of the first researchers in the Netherlands to report data related to bisexuality. His data comes from a national, representative sex survey carried out in 1968, sponsored by one of the main women's magazines of that time. For this study use has been made of personal interviewing. In this study sexual preference has not been assessed with the usual bipolar Kinsey scale, containing seven or five intermediate steps between exclusive heterosexuality and exclusive homosexuality. Apparently assuming a heterosexual preference, subjects were asked to what extent they felt physically attracted to persons of the same sex—emotional attraction was not yet *en vogue* at that time. Differences were found between married and unmarried men and women, more or less homosexual attraction being observed most frequently in unmarried men (14 percent) and less frequently in married men (2 percent). The married and unmarried women fell between these two extremes (respectively 9 percent and 4 percent).

Because in this survey one unipolar scale has been used, it is uncertain whether the persons who said that they feel somewhat or predominantly attracted to persons of their own sex were also attracted to persons of the other sex. Likewise it is unclear how many of these men and women would have labeled their preference as bisexual. The author was alarmed by the great number of married persons, and therefore presumably heterosexual, having homosexual attractions. He assumed this discrepancy to be a consequence of social pressures to live a heterosexual life. Furthermore he expected this discrepancy to have a negative influence on marital satisfaction. Unfortunately the survey did not show how these people expressed their sexuality, how they labeled their preference, how they designed their sexual and intimate lives, and what kind of problems they were confronted with.

More precise information comes from a national survey for which data have been collected in 1989 (n = 1,000; Van Zessen and Sandfort 1991). Because of AIDS it had become relevant at that time to ask more precisely about sexual preference and the sex of sex partners. In line with the spirit of the time, it was not assumed in the questionnaire that people were married or that they had a heterosexual preference. Using the Kinsey scale, only 0.5 percent of the women and none of the men chose the (bisexual) midpoint to describe their sexual attraction. With respect to sexual behavior in the preceding year, 1.9 percent of all the men in the sample and 0.5 percent of all the women could be classified as bisexual, meaning that they have had sexual contacts with men as well as with women in that year. Of the persons who had had sex with both men and women, most labeled themselves as exclusively or predominantly heterosexual.

Labeling one's sexual preference as "heterosexual as well as homosexual" does not necessarily imply that the person involved has a well-balanced, integrated sexual identity. This might be hindered partly by social pressures to choose between both preferences and the lack of available bisexual models. Generally, bisexuality is accepted neither by heterosexuals nor homosexuals, the first reproaching bisexuals for making the best of both worlds, and the latter accusing bisexuals of suppressing their true (homo)sexual feelings. The midpoint of the Kinsey scale might also have been chosen by some subjects to indicate that one still has not yet made up his or her mind. The persons who reported particular doubts about their sexual preference were the young ones who had placed themselves in the middle category.

With respect to the numbers of sex partners, persons with bisexual behavior in the past year take an exceptional position. Irrespective of the time frame—the preceding year, the preceding five years, or entire life—the mean number of partners of bisexual men is between that of exclusively heterosexual and exclusively homosexual men. For bisexual women, the mean number of partners is higher than that of heterosexual as well as of homosexual women. The figures coming from this as well as other studies are all based on self-reported behavior (Van Zessen and Sandfort 1991). This implies a certain reticence in drawing conclusions. Bisexuality being considered a form of deviant behavior, underreporting may have influenced the data. Using the same questionnaire as Van Zessen and Sandfort, Van Griensven (Veugelers et al. 1991) studied a representative group of men in the city of Amsterdam (N = 709), the city with most of the Dutch AIDS cases. Of the total sample, more men labeled themselves as "heterosexual as well as homosexual" than in the national sample (1.6 percent). Some of these men had had no sex in the preceding year; others had had sex with men or women. Surprisingly, none of the behaviorally bisexual men classified themselves as "heterosexual as well as homosexual." Unlike those in the national survey, bisexual men in this study had the highest number of partners in the preceding year. They also seemed to practice unsafe sexual behavior more often than heterosexual or homosexual men. Of these three groups, 60.0 percent, 20.7 percent, and 9.1 percent respectively had had unprotected vaginal or anal intercourse outside of a steady relationship.

LABELING

One might expect the prevalence of bisexual self-labeling to occur more often when one deals with selected groups, like gay men. In a postal survey among the readership of a national gay newspaper, 2 percent labeled their sexual preference as "heterosexual as well as homosexual" (Tielman and Polter 1986). Looking at marital status, a different picture arises: 2 percent of the men were currently married and 2 percent had been married but were divorced. Of course, being married does not necessarily imply sexual interaction. However, figures from a national sample suggest that there are almost no marriages in which no sexual contacts take place (Van Zessen and Sandfort 1991). The mean ages of the men in the married and the divorced groups are significantly higher than the age of the men who have never been married. This suggests that marriage as a refuge—with subsequent divorce—has become a less unavoidable stage in the development of a homosexual lifestyle. This will have been predominantly a consequence of the growing tolerance for homosexual behavior in the Netherlands (Van Naerssen and Schreurs 1991). The same study shows that of the 1,003 men who have been sexually active in the preceding half-year, 5.5 percent have had sexual contacts with men as well as with women in that period. This percentage is indeed higher then the one found in the national study, dealing with a period which is twice as long.

BISEXUALITY AND YOUTH

Figures about the prevalence of bisexual contacts in early youth are available from a retrospective study, carried out in the mid eighties among young people eighteen to twenty-three years old (Sandfort 1988, 1991). All together, 283 persons were interviewed; 175 of them from an a select sample of Dutch young people. The remaining 108 persons were selected because they had had, before the age of sixteen, voluntary as well as nonconsensual sexual experiences with adults. The sexual experiences with each partner these young people had had, were separately investigated. Compared with the figures of the national sample, a fair number of the respondents in the select group had sexual contacts with both sexes: 7.5 percent of the 53 men and 8.2 percent of the 49 women. This will partly be a consequence of a slightly broader definition of sexual contact used in the study among young adults. In the select group there are even more respondents who had sexual contacts with persons of the other as well as their own sex (51.6 percent of the 31 men and 11.7 percent of the 77 women).

Some of the respondents had severe nonconsensual experiences. Excluding these subjects from further analysis, it is possible to say something about the backgrounds and possible consequences of bisexual experiences, by comparing the bisexual respondents with respondents who have had sexual contacts only with persons of one sex. The backgrounds of both groups do not differ significantly. The social climate of the family in which they grew up has been the same for both groups. Likewise, the parents do not differ with respect to physical attention they have paid to their child as well as their sexual attitudes. Finally, there are no differences with respect to religious background. However, respondents with bisexual experiences started to masturbate at an earlier age than those without these experiences. In the study, onset of masturbation has been shown to be an indicator of sexual interest, implying that bisexual behavior in early youth might be caused by a stronger sexual interest.

With respect to sexual functioning in later life, the study shows some differences between the respondents with bisexual experiences and those with experiences with one sex only (again, leaving out the young people with severe, nonconsensual experiences). The first group has a stronger sexual desire and a lesser degree of sexual anxiety. One has to be careful in interpreting these relationships as causal. The differences may be a consequence of other factors as well; besides, retrospective distortion may have resulted in an artificial relation.

Some insights into the dynamics of bisexual behavior might be found in research carried out among young boys (between ten and sixteen years old) involved in pedophile relationships (Sandfort 1982, 1987). Although they are sexually involved with somebody of the same sex, they do not see themselves as gay. Nor do they label themselves as bisexual. Almost all of them, with one clear exception, see themselves as "straight," expecting to have sex with girls and to get married in the future. It seems that their sexual involvement and enjoyment of the "homo"-sexual contact should not be explained by the sexual attraction to the other male. As long as they do not have a receptive role, their excitement being caused by the sexual stimulation of the partner, being sexually active might itself be the source of sexual excitement. These findings warn us against the implicit assumption that sexual contacts are always based on feelings of (sexual) attraction to the other person. Especially with respect to bisexuality, this assumption of sexual attraction toward an object might impede a true understanding of the dynamics underlying this form of sexual behavior.

NEW INTEREST IN BISEXUALITY

A recent sign of the growing interest in bisexuality is the publication of a book dealing with the bisexual lives of 23 men and 23 women between the ages of 21 to 76, living in the Netherlands (Hanson 1990). Based on written questionnaires and personal interviews, the dilemmas of a bisexual lifestyle are illustrated. Almost all respondents seemed to long for relationships with a man and with a woman at the same time. This valuable, in-depth study probably shows, however, only a part of bisexual behavior of Dutch citizens, namely the behavior of those who label themselves as bisexual. The main purpose of this book seems to legitimize the bisexual experience and to further the construction of a bisexual identity. One should realize that most bisexual behavior will occur without being labeled as bisexual. In effect this category of persons is almost inaccessible to targeted prevention activities.

CONCLUSIONS

This overview shows that only little is known about bisexuality in the Netherlands. In-depth research is needed to assess the necessity of HIV prevention and to survey the possibilities of carrying out specific prevention activities effectively. To get a comprehensive overview of the different forms of bisexuality, one should realize that this form of behavior might be determined by personal factors as well as situational factors, or a combination of the two. Situational factors can play different roles. For example, they can result in making access to partners of the desired sex physically impossible. In this instance, it is interesting to find out why and how some men adjust their sexual attraction, while others don't, and how they deal with these experiences in terms of their sexual identity. Situational factors, like the general sexual climate in a society, may also postpone the development of homosexual attraction, and "force" people into heterosexual relationships, in which they unknowingly or consciously engage themselves. Among situational factors one should also consider the social norms which inhibit or prescribe bisexuality. This might be of special importance since Western European culture is becoming more and more a mixture of (sub)cultures.

Probably related to personal factors is the dimension of self-labeling, which puts the behavior in a new perspective. Related to both, that is, the personal as well as the situational factors, might be the viewpoint of sexual development: during adolescence, having sex with male as well as with female partners might be seen as a form of sexual openness, unrestricted by a limiting, sexual identity or as a willful experiment in the process of sexual identity formation. Although to a lesser extent than in former times, inaccessibility of girls is still a situational factor stimulating sexually precocious boys to engage in sexual contacts with persons of their own sex.

At this moment, the main purpose of the study of bisexuality should be to make an inventory of the different shapes in which bisexual behavior occurs and to describe the divergent dynamics of this form of sexual expression. Subsequently it will be possible to quantify specific information and to determine if any form of prevention should be developed to deal with specific forms of bisexual behavior.

7

Patterns of Bisexuality in Sub-Saharan Africa

Tade Akin Aina

INTRODUCTION

It is perhaps necessary to begin by stating that sexuality in any of its forms (bisexuality, heterosexuality, or homosexuality) has, to a great extent, not received much direct research attention in Sub-Saharan Africa. Except on very rare occasions, the little attention that has been paid to it has been subsumed under the broad areas of ethnographic or sociological accounts of kinship and marriage. This neglect is even greater in relation to the study of homosexuality and bisexuality. The urgency and scope for extensive research on the patterns of human sexuality in Sub-Saharan Africa, particularly in light of the current AIDS pandemic, are therefore great. Also, a focus on bisexuality and homosexuality is further complicated by the nature of the overt conventional response to the phenomenon by Africans in general, which is often fright, confusion, and denial of such forms of sexuality.

An understanding of the pattern of bisexuality in Africa cannot be complete without an understanding of the different factors that have come to determine the values and practice of sex that are held in African societies. These factors include (a) traditional African conceptions of sexuality; (b) the fact of external contacts and its implications for sexual practices, attitudes, and values; and (c) the more recent impact of modernization and affluence on social behavior and their implications for sexual norms and practices. All these influence the way in which bisexuality is treated here. In this chapter an analysis is made of this pattern in the context of its implications for the emerging AIDS epidemic, the threat posed by it, and the prejudice and fear that have accompanied it.

It is argued here that while bisexuality was not nonexistent in precolonial Africa, it was never really open to all, nor understood by all. Male bisexuality was practiced by a minority in relation to either ritualistic needs or as an institutionalized adjustment and tension-management device. Female bisexuality, on the other hand, was seen in terms of pleasure-seeking activity but not considered a problem. External contact with Europe and the Arab world further generalized and strengthened the existence of male homosexual relations. Inasmuch as most of the African participants were not exclusively homosexual, such sexual orientation was in essence bisexual.

Before proceeding further, a point of clarification is necessary here and that is that the coverage of Sub-Saharan Africa should be seen in its most general terms. The region is a massive, complex, and plural entity in terms of cultures, histories, and contemporary levels of socioeconomic development. A detailed treatment of her diversity cannot be carried out within the limits of a contribution such as this. What is attempted here is an examination based on evidence from history, ethnography, folklore, and contemporary observations. These are used to discuss the main patterns of bisexuality in Africa in precolonial, colonial, and contemporary times and to extract their implications for the AIDS pandemic.

Bisexuality in Precolonial Africa

Available evidence in the ethnographic literature, oral traditions, and folklore points to the existence of various forms of bisexual orientations and practices in precolonial Africa. Apart from the existence of ritual bisexuality, which is a special form of bisexual relations, there is also evidence of other forms of bisexual behavior such as situational bisexuality, bisexuality among married persons, adolescent bisexuality, and female bisexuality. The instances and patterns of these in precolonial Africa are further examined below.

Ritual Bisexuality

Ritual bisexuality was an aspect of a whole class of sexual relations related to the gaining of mystical powers and witchcraft. It involved, in the main, sexual activities that are considered deviant or sexual intercourse with odious or very unattractive partners such as, mainly, destitutes, the mentally ill, and partners who are seriously physically disabled and repulsive. The rationale behind this is that through this interaction the normal dominant partner draws from his less fortunate partner the predestined store or essence of good fortune and fate that all human beings are supposed to possess spiritually. In the case of ritual bisexuality that involves anal intercourse, it is believed by some groups in Africa, namely the Yorubas and Hausas of Nigeria, that through actual sexual intercourse the dominant partner augments and/or charges like a battery his own store of such quality or essence, thereby contributing to his increased success in whatever endeavors he undertakes. This ritual element thus contains a specific pattern of bisexual behavior.

Other Forms of Bisexuality

The second class of practices is that which was oriented toward the management of sexual tensions and an institutionalization of nonheterosexual relations among males. The patterns manifested in this class include examples of situational bisexuality, bisexuality among married persons, and adolescent bisexuality. These experiences in precolonial Africa have been documented by E. E. Evans-Pritchard, the famous British anthropologist, in his book on sexual and gender relations among the Azande of Sudan titled *Man and Woman Among the Azande*. Evans-Pritchard hinted at adolescent bisexuality and situational bisexuality when he discussed the phenomenon he called "marriage with boys." He pointed out the situational aspect of the relationship by showing that "marriage with boys" occurs because in the majority of cases, such men do not as yet possess legal access to women. Because of the heavy sanctions against having illegal access to women (such as mutilation of the genitals), some men practice marriage with boys: ". . . so for that reason a man used to marry a boy to have orgasm between his thighs which quieted the desire for a woman" (Evans-Pritchard 1974:37). Securing these rights of access to boys was a formal arrangement between families. Bridewealth of between five to ten spears was paid and if the man was "good" to his "in-laws," he was then given a girl to marry. The rationale was "good for a boy how much better for a woman" (Evans-Pritchard 1974:37). Another noteworthy aspect of the work is the statement of the cultural recognition of the need for bisexual relations among the Azande. Evans-Pritchard referred to men who "although they had (female) wives, still married boys" (Evans-Pritchard 1974:37). Other cases of bisexual behavior described in the study included female bisexuality and are examined under the title "lesbianism" (Evans-Pritchard 1974:122–25).

However, an important point that emerges from Evans-Pritchard's account is that although male bisexual relations constitute the essence of "marriage to boys" among the Azande, there is no evidence of anal intercourse. The closest reference to actual sexual contact are "orgasm between [the boy's] thighs." In a text that explicitly discusses sexual behavior such as autoeroticism, lesbianism, and heterosexual intercourse in other parts, it is to be assumed that this sentence literally means what it says.

What eventually happened to this indigenous institution and practice and what remains of it among the Azande are not available to us in any documented form. But if colonization and external contacts did drive this and other similar practices and institutions underground, it brought with it its own forms of bisexual relations, albeit in more alienated, more instrumental, and less effectively institutionalized modes.

EXTERNAL CONTACTS, COLONIZATION, AND BISEXUALITY IN AFRICA

Africa's external contacts, particularly with North Africa and the Middle East, date back several hundred years. The contact based on trade, religion, and later on conquest involved contacts with North Africa and the Middle East by West Africans via the Sahara desert, and contacts with North Africa and the Middle East (particularly Oman) with East and Central Africans via the Indian Ocean and the River Nile. The important aspect of the contact with Middle Eastern culture was the spread of the practice of male bisexual interaction. This, of course, occurred mainly in the tiny enclaves in which the aliens from the Arab world often stayed and consisted mainly of interactions either with the children of the aristocracy of such societies with whom they had very intense contacts as teachers or warders, or with eunuchs (an aspect of the culture), their other servants and slaves, and other clients. Although direct documented evidence of these activities, particularly in Sub-

Saharan Africa, is hard to come by, local folklore and oral traditions in parts of Nigeria, Cameroon, and Senegal in West Africa, and Kenya, Tanzania, and Uganda in East Africa, abound with insinuations, veiled references, and occasional blunt descriptions of this pattern of sexuality. The predominant forms are situational bisexuality among married persons, although ritual elements also emerge at times.

Colonization represented another mode of African contact with the outside world. Involving actual conquest, domination, and settlement, it had far-reaching implications for the transformation of societal institutions, beliefs, and social and cultural values. Colonization generated urbanization, industrialization, and modernization. It allowed greater anonymity, lesser integration with primordial institutions, and wider exposure and access to varied forms of sexual relations including those defined as unconventional by traditional society.

Colonization also expanded monetization and commercialization, including that of sex. Prostitution, in particular heterosexual prostitution, grew and developed during this period. Colonization also introduced institutions and contexts of prolonged single-sex settings within which bisexual culture and relations could thrive. These settings included the armed forces, the prison system, the single-sex boarding schools. In these places, the managers and administrators, particularly the British, brought with them single-sex norms and values of their middle class and aristocracy, including that of male homosexuality, that were widely available and acceptable in their own public schools and military barracks. Forms of bisexuality engaged in included adolescent bisexuality, bisexuality among married persons, and secondary homosexuality. However, it should be remembered that precolonial fears about homosexual sex coupled with the impact of the newly introduced Christian religion contributed to ensuring that bisexual interaction remained hidden by its practitioners, feared and hated by others, and unknown to many.

AFFLUENCE, EXPOSURE, AND MALE HOMOSEXUAL PROSTITUTION IN THE POSTCOLONIAL PERIOD

The postcolonial period witnessed a further increase in urbanization, the extension of modernization, the increase in the breakdown of traditional norms, and a new affluence. This new affluence, of course, did not benefit everybody. Its beneficiaries among the indigenous population were tiny minorities who were well enough placed to take advantage of the changes occasioned by decolonization of many of these countries in the 1960s.

This affluence occurred along with the more intense and increasing poverty of the vast majority of the ordinary peoples. The economic crisis, together with the ecological and political disasters that emerged, made matters worse for both the rural and urban poor and increased their vulnerability.

Africa's postcolonial affluence was also significant in the way it affected sexual values and mores. Its major aspect was that the affluent middle classes were in the main either much traveled or already exposed to Western and other influences.

In the realm of sexual behavior, affluence therefore brought about increasing "promiscuity" in sexual relations and an extensive commercialization both in terms of prostitution and another pool of "nonprofessional" practitioners who got involved in sexual relations mainly for material gratification. These often involved participants who did not actually demand money for sex, yet had partners who in return kept them, provided them with jobs, cheap consumer goods and, in some cases, expensive luxury goods, paid vacations, and entertainment.

This "pool," which can be found in virtually all major African cities, constituted the main ingredient of the "sugar-daddy" arrangement and serviced as it were the new-rich indigenes, the already wealthy white expatriates, the Asian and Levantine settlers, and the rapidly increasing tourist community. The "sugar-daddy arrangement" is a term used to describe liaisons between predominantly wealthier and older men and younger girls, who entered this mainly for the material benefits they could get. It operates along a continuum that includes elements of concubinage at one end, and the freest liaison at the other end. Central to it, however, is the disparity in age and social and economic status of the participants and the fact of material and other rewards.

These same processes occurred with male homosexual practices. Postcolonial affluence increased and expanded the dimensions of the phenomenon of male homosexual prostitution that had already been developing gradually since the colonial era. These prostitutes can be found in virtually all large African cities and tourist centers, around the five-star and other hotels catering mainly to an expatriate clientele and the local rich. In Nairobi, Lusaka, Dakar, Banjul, Abidjan, Lagos, Kaduna, and Kano, these prostitutes exist with their unique styles of soliciting and identifying potential customers. Often they double as pimps procuring female prostitutes for heterosexual relations; when there are clients interested in men they offer themselves. Interestingly enough, large numbers of these male prostitutes are bisexual. In fact, when not on business, some of them have confessed preference for heterosexual relations. Others have confessed that it has taken them quite some time— some about eight years—before they have become exclusively homosexual (*Prime People* 1988:5).

Apart from the male homosexual prostitution network that services what can be called an expatriate and tourist sector, there are also instances in Africa of an emerging predominantly indigenous sector. This is vividly illustrated by the northern Nigerian experience particularly in Kano, Kaduna, and some other cities. It is termed the *Dan-Daudu* phenomenon. According to Richard Umaru (1987):

> By the 1940s many of these boys had completed their "homosexual tutelage," [and] set up businesses in most northern urban centers as full-time professional homosexuals. This is the origin of the Hausa institution of *Dan Daudu*. *Yan Daudus* (plural of Dan Daudu) are men who dress in women's clothes, talk like women, cook and sell food, and generally run brothels from whence both male and female prostitutes can be obtained on payment of a commission. However, the male prostitutes carry out their business secretly and discreetly. . . . Indeed the Yan Daudus play the dual role of procuring clients as well as training young boys and girls who ran away from their homes (mainly child-brides) in prostitution.

As can be inferred from the above, the Yan Daudus are male homosexual prostitutes who compete with female prostitutes in the red-light districts to solicit for customers. These are mainly a crop of low-income young urban dwellers or migrants who have moved into this business mainly for reasons of keeping body and soul together. They approximate to Ross's (1989) categorization of secondary homosexuality. These men, although not as aggressive and obvious as the female heterosexual prostitutes, are available and identifiable by their styles and demeanor in the streets that constitute the red-light district of the Sabon-Gari area of Kano. Their clientele consists predominantly of wealthy members of the commercial, bureaucratic, and professional elites. The prostitutes have also developed an intricate system of bargaining and liaison with their clientele.

Apart from outright prostitution, the "sugar-daddy arrangement" is also used in male homosexual relationships in some countries, such as Nigeria, for instance. This includes a more or less stable relationship between partners of unequal economic means. Again for the poorer partner, there is an instrumentalist motive as material and other benefits are derived from the relationship. This sort of arrangement has been found quite attractive by several young men, and it increasingly becomes a means of mobility and acquisition of wealth.

Another aspect of this phenomenon, though, is concubinage. The "sugar-daddies" themselves often operate plural relationships with a retinue of young men who are of course regularly rewarded for their services. Again, both the "sugar-daddies" and their friends tend to be bisexual. In fact, most of the younger men tend to utilize resources derived from their homosexual relations in pursuing aggressive hetero-sexual activities. They are often identifiable as big spenders and playboy socialites.

Still tied up, however, with the practice of male homosexuality are some elements of the precolonial beliefs about nonconventional sexuality. Even the male homosexual prostitutes interviewed in Kano and Lagos in Nigeria still believe that there are magical and witchcraft effects asso-ciated with male homosexual intercourse. They also believe that if the dominant partner is a businessman, such associations confer spiritual benefits to his business. This, they state, affects the price they place on their services. Also it is felt that homosexuality conveys some unique advantages on its practitioners; for instance, they feel that homosexuals tend to be rich and successful men. Tied up with this is the perception of risks. The prostitutes interviewed feel that they are at risk of becoming impotent (the "eunuch effect") or permanently incapable of conventional heterosexual relations once any of their clients exploit the relationship either for ritual or witchcraft purposes. Thus mentally, there is still the combination of instrumentalist and material needs alongside the pre-colonial perceptions of the benefits and dangers of nonconventional sex-ual practices. Among the Nigerian prostitutes spoken to, modern risks such as AIDS or sexually transmitted diseases did not carry weight as sources of fear. There was neither a great fear nor serious recognition of the risks these posed.

IGNORANCE, PREJUDICE, AND HIV RISKS IN SUB-SAHARAN AFRICA

The first point that requires attention in the campaign on AIDS in Africa is that commercial consideration more than hedonism is a major element of the growth of male homosexual prostitution. From all indications, particularly with the protracted current economic crisis in Africa, male homosexual prostitution will continue to grow as a form of seeking a living.

Secondly, there is the fact that many of the practitioners are bisexual. In fact, many of those involved in what we have called the "sugar-daddy arrangement" have demonstrated an overt inclination for aggressive and multiple, simultaneous heterosexual relations.

Finally, there is still too much ignorance about the risks of AIDS and other sexually transmitted diseases even among male homosexual prostitutes. From a few focus-group interviews held in Lagos and Kano, what seems to emerge is very little fear of disease and more fear of witchcraft, persecution, and prosecution. This is in spite of the growing number of HIV cases in the continent.

The implications of all of this is that both AIDS and other sexually transmitted diseases can be transmitted simultaneously through homosexual and heterosexual means by the same groups of persons. There is, therefore, the need for a systematic and extensive public-enlightenment campaign. This, however, requires sensitive and sympathetic handling, rather than the fomentation of dubious moral and religious sentiments or trivial sensationalization by the mass media. Already, the trends in the media coverage of male homosexual practices possess strong elements of prejudice both in the choice of key words and reportorial slant. In societies where nonconventional sexual practices are surrounded by a haze of mystical and witchcraft beliefs, fears, and suspicion, the consequences of a negative and prejudiced mass reaction cannot be underestimated. There is the need for great care in this regard not only to avoid promoting a situation of mass hysteria and persecution of Africa's increasing number of male bisexuals but, more seriously, to avoid driving underground a larger group of erstwhile male homosexual prostitutes and sugar-daddy partners who, though they engage in the act for its rewards, are themselves bisexual.

More extensive research to document the social conditions, lifestyles, and situations of male homosexual prostitutes, their clients, and female partners is urgently required if the information necessary for devising an effective strategy and plan of action is to be obtained.

IMPLICATIONS FOR AIDS PREVENTION

What the discussions above show is the clear-cut existence of bisexual relations and practice in Sub-Saharan Africa over different periods. It also shows the recent expansion of the commercialization of sex through prostitution, particularly male homosexual prostitution. The prostitutes themselves are involved in what has been termed secondary homosexuality. They are therefore predominantly bisexual, engaging simultaneously in relationships with both female and male partners. Because of the high turnover of partners in their professional activities and the very nature of their sexual interaction, these subjects are engaged in high-risk behavior in regard to contracting and spreading of HIV. There is, therefore, the greatest need and urgency to promote safe-sex attitudes among them. This is limited, however, by the fact that very little or no systematic research exists with regard to who they are, who their partners are, who their clients are, the patterns of their sexual lives, their fears, and the social and health risks to which they are exposed. Such knowledge is an essential component of any successful campaign to combat AIDS.

8

Patterns of Bisexuality in India

Bhushan Kumar

Biologically a human being is not purely unisexual. Sexual pleasure is obviously a crucial matrix binding all sexual behavior. Freud (1925) contended that all human beings combine in themselves both masculine and feminine characteristics. As stated by Virginia Woolf, "it is fatal to be a man or woman pure and simple: one must be woman-manly or man-womanly."

The concept of bisexuality has its origins in folklore and mythology. It was believed that a human being is behaviorally bisexual at birth and that the final pattern of sexual behavior depends on later environmental influences (Ellenberger 1970). Heilbrun (1973) stated that our future salvation lies in a movement away from sexual polarization. A statement of bisexuality means that one is seen as a heterosexual who has gay affairs, and not the other way around. Bisexual behavior occurs only in human beings and not in animals except in certain exceptional situations. A few homosexual men indeed may have families without giving up homosexuality entirely. This form of homosexuality does not cancel out the heterosexual desires, although sex with a partner of the same sex may be more enjoyable. Humphreys (1970), though, made mention of a considerable number of married men who regularly had homosexual contacts but could not define the mechanisms at work, giving fluidity to the term bisexuality (Herdt 1985).

Anthropologically and historically Cypriot, Greek, Egyptian (Isis-Osiris), Japanese (Izanami-Izanagi), and many Arab, Mexican, and Hebrew doctrines describe their divinities as bisexual (Bhattacharya 1978). The Greek story of Tiresias, the male seer who spent seven years as a woman, is probably the best known of many legends depicting men and women who changed sex during the course of their lives. There are traces of bisexuality in the Old Testament and certain Egyptian gods were notoriously bisexual (Bancroft 1983). Julius Caesar's diversity of sexual tastes earned him the reputation of being "the husband of every woman and the wife of every man," but even Caesar was scandalized by the harem of both sexes Mark Antony kept in Rome.

After noting a few facts from other parts of the world, from the sociologists and anthropologists, it seems to be useful at the outset to try to analyze sex life on the subcontinent of India in past ages to form a basis for understanding less common sexual practices in India. The Hindu concept of full life postulates the harmony of three activities: *dharma* (morality), *artha* (polity), and *kama* (love and sex). In Rigveda (2500 B.C.) they say that it was not unusual to separate and seclude women from men. The *purdah* (veil or a curtain) to screen women from the sight of strangers (men) was in vogue. In the epics of Mahabharta and Ramayana (between 600 and 200 B.C.) there are references to privacy and isolation of women (Shah 1961). Manu (a great Indian sage, 200 B.C.) forbade the mingling of women with men. *Kamasutra* (Indian treatise on love), the monumental work of Vatsayana (200 B.C. to 500 A.D.), mentions at least seven different types of kissing, eight varieties of touching, etc. During its discussions of love making, there is also a mention of homosexuality in very derogatory and degrading terms, but there is no mention of bisexuality. Manu in *Manu-Smriti* (a book on social code, 200 A.D.) discusses punishments to be meted out to homosexual men and women and those engaging in "sexual perversions." The South Indian book on ethics (*Thirukural,* 200 A.D.) is against homosexuality (Somasundaram 1986). Anal intercourse was only to be practiced with a woman to degrade and humiliate her. Homosexual and heterosexual oral genital sex has been mentioned and grudgingly licensed in special situations. The work of Vatsayana left its deep impressions on art. The *maithuna* or the union (mating) sculptures are to be found in the temples of Konarak, Khajuraho, Belur, and Halebidu. Such scenes are also found in the Buddhist paintings at Nagarjunikonda and Ajanta and Jain temples. In temples of Khajuraho (850–1050 A.D.) there is a statue showing a woman in a standing position, engaged in sex with two men, one using the vaginal and the other the anal orifice.

Hindu legends, art, and literature refer to homosexuality and bisexuality, but Hinduism as a religion is not very informative on the subject. There is a mention of the many paired deities from the time of Rig Vedas, the most notable being Ardhanarisvara (the half-male and half-female figure of the God Shiva) (Sinha 1966). In a legend in the Rig Vedas, Yama was conceived as having the character of a hermaphrodite. Afterward, he was split into Yama and Yami, a male and a female who were regarded as the first parents of human beings (Dandekar 1962). So the pair is just one single, undivided entity, self-cloven into two halves for the sake of creation. The Upanishads explain the course of creation by the principle of duality. Prajapati (the creator), tired of solitude, produces the world after having divided himself in two: a male half and a female half. The Samkhya cosmology also propounds a similar theory of creation. And the theory recurs in many *Puranas* (highly valued socioreligious books) (Banerjea 1956). The statue of Natraja is also considered as a form of Ardhanarisvara. The religion in the *Puranas* developed the concept of an androgynous god, and we find in the Hindu pantheon many androgynous deities (also to stress the important and equal status of women) (Banerjea 1956). The Tantric (a cult) and Buddhists have accepted and propagated the principle of dualism in the absolute oneness. The Chinese conceived the twin principles of Yin (female) and Yang (male) for creation. All this points out that each of us is an Ardhanarisvara who aspires to resolve the paradox of the opposite into unity, not by negation but through positive experiences of life. Therefore, out of inescapable logic we may accept the relevancy of the prospect of bisexuality as a fundamental fact. The bisexuality mentioned above is a perspective of real vision, a perspective for understanding the totality of humanity biologically, psychologically, and sociologically. This perspective of bisexuality has deep relevance in understanding the human being in distress.

Indeed in the world today, heterosexual intercourse is the preferred mode of self-expression for most adults, but some do engage in other forms of sexual behavior as well.

Manifest sexual behavior is intertwined with social, cultural, religious, and moral values of the society. Apart from the self-identified (contingent invert) homosexuals, there are those situational (amphigenic invert) homosexuals who take to homosexuality on odd occasions or when suitable heterosexual partners are not available. This is especially true for Indian society that stresses virginity tremendously. The same may happen to someone who is forcibly deprived of contact with the opposite sex, for instance, during imprisonment, in hostels, or in segregated boarding schools. It is an easy way out, especially for those in authority like the jail warders, teachers, and wardens in hostels and reformatories. So homosexuality may be an acknowledged way of life because of protracted segregation of sexes. There was an interesting observation made by Dr. Upjeet Kaur (personal communication) who, while trying to find out the incidence of sexual transmissibility of the hepatitis-B virus, was inquiring into the sexual habits of adult males from North India. Thirty-one of the 1,311 men avowed that they engaged in same-gender sexual relationships. It was revealed by 15 of these 31 homosexuals that they would prefer to go to a female prostitute for heterosexual sex if they had enough money but had to be content with homosexuality for want of enough pocket allowance, thus adding another class to the group of situational homosexuals. So these situational homosexuals use the same-gender sexual relationship only as a convenient substitute (for want of money), without its interfering with their preferred heterosexual capacity or feeling. These bisexuals are probably able to find full erotic satisfaction with those of either sex.

Bisexuals usually claim a permanent need for concurrent relations with both sexes to enjoy the best of both worlds, as it were. Because of their dual orientation, they may sometimes exhibit conflicts over their ambivalent personality and may tend to tilt more toward one type of sexual behavior under various modifying social conditions and states of psychological well-being. They would be classified in the middle range of Kinsey's homosexual-heterosexual scale. It seems natural that some males may be involved in both homosexual and heterosexual practices simultaneously, concurrently, or serially. It may also be that, as in some other societies, the inserter male does not conceptualize himself as a homosexual, as is the case, for example, with Mestizo Mexicans (Carrier 1985).

Many Indian men and others in a traditional society may have to maintain a bisexual life because they are trapped in marriage obligations, continue to need the security and support of a home life, or remain unwilling to accept for themselves the still onerous identity of being homosexual. Moreover, if we believe that biologically we are either homosexual or heterosexual, then those who mingle the two "become cowards and losers and are viewed with suspicion and intolerance" (Paul 1984). Who would like to dare? Devi (1977), after interviewing many Indian homosexual men, noted that marriage is considered a duty and obligation to one's family rather than an expression of individual sexual preference. Freund et al. (1982) suggested that bisexual identity may be claimed by homosexuals because of the stigmatization of homosexuality.

In some situations sex in the Hindu society has acquired religious overtones. It is there treated with reserve and the rules have to be solemnly complied with.

Because of this, the ancient Hindus were divided into two groups: the licentious and self-indulgent constituting one category, and the renunciators of the flesh and the world the other. Even the first group rigidly adhered to the doctrine that the "right kind" of sexual contact was only permissible in wedlock. Like all known cultures, Hindu philosophy (literature and scriptures) is in favor of copulation between men and women, as contrasted with alternative avenues of sexual expression, because society cannot favor a nonproductive form of sexual activity if it wants to save itself from extinction. This is also stated in the "common-sense theory" by Davenport (1977). However, the greater emphasis on individualism due to modernization, individual social stresses, education, economic freedom, and social acceptance of divorce combined with Western materialistic influence and resultant greater sexual freedom has demystified sex. Personal choice seems to be becoming more important, though only to a small number of people. For most people collective society has supremacy over the individual (sexually liberated or not), and sexual behavior should conform to rigid and strong social norms.

Transsexualism in India is uncommon (Shrivastava et al. 1985). Eunuchs (hermaphrodites) often act as passive partners during same-sex sexual activities. Their number was roughly over one million at the last count (Sharma 1989).

Nakra et al. (1978), in a study of the sexual behavior of the north Indian male, found no history of bisexuality in the 150 men interviewed.

Bisexuals, at least in India, seem to be at the moment very much between the devil and the deep blue sea. This is as a consequence of the confusion created and perpetuated by the rigidly, advocated and expected sexual behavior and not so clearly defined views in old Indian art and culture. In the absence of unequivocal scientific criteria of bisexual behavior, it may be deemed pathological because it contrasts with the mores and behavior of a dichotomous society. Biology is neutral on the subject; history, anthropology, art, and religion provide conflicting evidence across time.

In our cross-cultural study (Kumar and Ross 1990) on 44 north

Indian homosexual men, most men had had bisexual experiences in the past two months. Half of the men were married, emphasizing marriage and lack of a distinct homosexual subculture in India. It was noteworthy that a quarter of them engaged in heterosexual anal sex. This may rapidly blur the distinction between the homosexual and heterosexual transmission of HIV. The lack of the Indian male's knowledge about the prophylactic value of condoms as reported by Jeyasingh et al. (1986) worsens things. So the situational Indian homosexual male has a tendency to revert quickly to heterosexual sex. This bisexual behavior will make difficult the identification of the at-risk groups for spread of HIV infection.

Bisexuality is a common enough phenomenon. But when a subject is highly controversial and especially if it involves sex, one cannot be expected to tell the whole truth. In Indian society, sex has been a taboo topic and hence has not been subjected to proper investigation. In the absence of any scientific and detailed study of contemporary attitudes or behavior, people generally base their views on speculation and make unscientific generalizations.

9

Patterns of Bisexuality in Thailand*

Wiresit Sittitrai, Tim Brown, and Sirapone Virulrak

INTRODUCTION

This chapter attempts to describe bisexuality as it occurs in Thailand. First, the existence and meaning of bisexuality in the Thai social context will be discussed, followed by a description of the patterns of bisexuality observed. Basic implications of these behaviors for the spread of HIV in the country are then laid out, followed by a discussion of future research needs to allow for the development of effective interventions targeting bisexual individuals. At present, available research material on the subject of Thai bisexuality is extremely limited. For this report, the primary sources of information are self-reports as published in various Thai gay magazines, existing survey data, in-depth interviews with key informants, and observations in various community settings in both Bangkok and other provinces.

---

*Data collection for this study was conducted by Dr. Sittitrai and his staff and funded by the Program on AIDS, Thai Red Cross Society. The Survey on Partner Relations and Risk of HIV Infection in Thailand was conducted by the Program on AIDS, Thai Red Cross Society and the Institute of Population Studies, Chulalongkorn University in 1990 and was funded by the Global Programme on AIDS of the World Health Organization.

OPENING REMARKS

Before beginning, we would like to spend a few moments outlining some of the difficulties that must be kept in mind in discussing the term "bisexuality." Bisexuality can be taken in several ways. First, it may be used as a description of sexual experience or behaviors on the part of an individual, i.e., as a description of a person who has sex with members of both sexes during some arbitrary period of time. It can also be used as a description of the person's underlying preference for sexual partners, i.e., that the person finds sexual encounters with either sex to be sexually exciting and generally prefers having sex with both men and women to having it exclusively with one sex. It can further be taken as a term of self-identification, that the person sees himself/herself as desiring or engaging in sexual encounters with members of both sexes. A final definition of "bisexuality" comes at the societal level, i.e., what other members of the society perceive as a "bisexual." For example, in some societies a married effeminate man might be viewed and regarded societally as bisexual regardless of his own behavior, preference, or self-identification.

Any single individual may be described as fitting any one of these frames of reference for "bisexuality" without fitting into the others. For example, in Thailand the majority of male bar workers definitely engage in sexual intercourse with both men and women but actually prefer having sex with women and would describe themselves as heterosexual in orientation, i.e., their behavior is bisexual, their preference is heterosexual, they self-identify as heterosexuals, and society sees them as homosexual or bisexual. They choose to have homosexual encounters out of a profit motive.

The issue of societal perceptions of bisexuality can become very complex, with different portions of the population seeing bisexuality in a different light. For example, in general Thai society, bisexuality is considered more acceptable than homosexuality, so many men with homosexual orientations might prefer to be labeled bisexual. Gay men in Thailand tend to find bisexuals and straights more attractive than other gay men. This may be illustrative of the perception that they are "harder to get" than gay men, that many Thai gay men perceive themselves as being more feminine in nature and find the masculinity attractive, or that bisexual and straight men are thought to be better in bed, especially if the gay man prefers anal-receptive intercourse.

A final group whose perceptions of bisexuality are critical in the context of HIV transmission is the epidemiologists, and through them the medical establishment and the public. The most common perception of bisexuals by epidemiologists is as a "risk group" that may serve as a bridge between different segments of the population. From a public health-planning point of view, this is a useful concept, especially in terms of providing targets for prevention efforts designed to reach those individuals whose behaviors place them at the highest risk of HIV transmission. But when this concept is conveyed to the public, it results in what the authors will label "risk-group syndrome."

In "risk-group syndrome," the term "risk groups" is presented to the public, generally through the popular media. The picture presented implies that if you are not a member of a risk group, you need not be concerned about AIDS/HIV. In receiving only a limited definition of "risk groups" without full information on risk behaviors, an individual may then easily avoid self-identification as a member of existing risk groups, regardless of the actual level of risk behavior. What many believe to be a good concept for those targeting interventions now becomes a dangerous misconception in the public mind. Given the human propensity for self-identifying out of any group perceived as a social problem, most individuals, even those engaging in high levels of risk behaviors, will not identify themselves as being members of any risk group and will continue to engage in risk behaviors.

An example of this was seen in Thailand two to three years ago, where the media initially presented the AIDS epidemic as a problem of only gay and intravenous drug-using groups with a strong emphasis on "foreigners" (*farang* in Thai), particularly Americans, as sources of HIV. This presentation of the problem had several serious consequences for the spread of HIV in Thailand. From the point of view of gay men, this media image was probably a positive factor in sensitizing them to the issue, and apparently it has resulted in behavioral change, as evidenced by the comparatively low prevalence of HIV in gay populations in Thailand.

Unfortunately, the media image gave the incorrect impression that heterosexuals had nothing to worry about. People were not concerned about the possibility that heterosexual spread, especially to and from the large population of female sex workers, would become the most rapidly growing form of HIV transmission in the country today. This can be seen from the statement of one man who tested HIV positive at the Thai Red Cross Clinic: "How can I get AIDS? I never had sex with men. I am not a gay."

In the early stages of the epidemic, this simplified version of the facts led to a separation between "Thai" gay bars and "farang" gay bars. In the "Thai" bars there were no "farang" admitted under the assumption that since "farang" were the source of HIV, there could be no HIV transmission between Thais. This meant that few safer-sex precautions were taken at these bars even long after the infected Thais in the country far outnumbered the infected foreigners who might be present. Some Thai gay men incorrectly seized on the "American" as the sole source of HIV. As one gay man said: "I don't have to worry, I only have sex with Europeans."

As the above examples illustrate, humans seem to have the ability always to see themselves as not at risk, especially when operating with limited knowledge. But this is not the only problem with "risk group" presentations; they also carry inertia. The public has a long memory, and even after epidemiologists in Thailand realized that the epidemic was not following the Western pattern, the images of gay and IVDU (intravenous drug user) risk groups persist in the public mind. Although there are attempts being made now to focus attention on risk behaviors, for example, by informing the public of the need for taking precautions in heterosexual contacts, it will take time to reverse the initial perceptions of limited "risk groups." Like many medical problems, "risk-group syndrome" lingers for a long time and continues to take its toll in continued risk behaviors and HIV transmission.

This concept must be remembered when discussing bisexuality in Thailand. It must be remembered that what is important here is risk behaviors, not risk groups. If the picture is painted of bisexuals as a major risk group, people will find personal justifications for placing themselves outside of this group rather than altering their behaviors. If the emphasis is placed on risk behaviors, however, stressing the risk in both heterosexual and homosexual encounters with infected partners, it will be more difficult for people to avoid recognizing their own risk. Those working in AIDS prevention would do well to remember this when communicating with the media. While concepts of risk groups may be easier to explain to reporters and the general public than risk behaviors, they generally create long-lasting misconceptions that may set back prevention efforts by years.

With the issues discussed in this section in mind, the following discussion will be framed primarily in terms of bisexual behavior. For purposes of this chapter, a functional definition of a bisexual as one who engages in sexual interactions with members of both sexes will be used. This is the most germane definition when addressing issues of HIV transmission; however, when dealing with interventions with individuals exhibiting bisexual behavior, issues of self-identification, preference, and societal perception become important.

SOCIO-CULTURAL CONTEXT

Thailand is situated in Southeast Asia with a population of 56 million people, approximately 20 percent of whom live in urban areas. The largest city is Bangkok with a population of 9 million, and the country is divided into four regions. Ranked from largest to smallest in terms of population, they are the Northeast, Central, North, and South. There are distinctive regional variations in terms of dialect and subculture, but there is a strong national identity, with the Central dialect being taught and understood in all regions. This sense of national identity is strengthened by good mass-media communications and a reliable transportation network reaching almost everywhere in the country. In the last two decades urbanization has been rapid, with towns becoming cities and the cities subsequently expanding in size. This has happened in each region; examples are Chiangmai, Khon Kaen, and Phuket. Notable characteristics include Westernization of lifestyle (encouraged by the importation of Western movies, music, and television), rapid expansion of the tourist trade, industrialization related to agriculture and garments, immigration into the cities from rural areas, and widespread development of sexual-service industries. In terms of sexual opportunity, larger cities offer not only convenient places for individuals to meet and locations for casual sexual contacts, but also the anonymity of being able to move about freely without the feeling that one's actions are known to one's neighbors, as in small towns or villages.

In terms of socio-economic and cultural contexts, the status of women in Thailand has always been higher than in other countries in Asia. When compared to women's position before the turn of the century, the status of Thai women has been improving. Women can now continue on to higher education and are attaining high political and business ranks. The usual norms are that women control the finances of the household and that many of the important decisions in the households are shared by the husband and wife. Despite this, the general norms of sexual expression for women are still limited, although more open than in some other societies, while men have few limitations in terms of sexual freedom. Thailand is known for its culture of permissiveness, in which the existence of norms and guidelines for behavior is rarely accompanied by serious social sanctions for their violation. The dominant Buddhist religion and the traditional Thai personality contribute to the existence of liberal values and attitudes in general.

The recent rapid modernization in conjunction with these traditional attitudes has resulted in changes in patterns and norms concerning courtship, freedom in mate-selection, lessened importance of virginity and marriage in the popular perception, and decrease in age of first intercourse. It has also led to more open discussion of sexual matters among certain groups of the population. It is likely that different patterns of sexual preference have existed in Thailand for some time, but only recently have they been expressed more openly. In this context, the expansion of tourism, the increased availability of various forms of commercial sex both for men and women and for locals and tourists, and the increased openness of sexuality are all interrelated (Sittitrai and Barry 1991).

SOCIAL IMAGES OF GENDER/FACTORS AFFECTING SEXUALITY

Before beginning the discussion of current patterns of bisexuality in Thailand, it is worth noting that many Western concepts of gender (perceived appearance and identification of sexual orientation) and rules of social interaction within and between the sexes do not apply. In this section some of these issues are outlined to set the stage for a discussion of the forms of bisexuality in Thailand.

In discussing bisexuality in Thai society, it is necessary to realize that male/female differences in appearance have not always been perceived to be as great as in Western societies. In fact, one must inquire whether the social images of males and females that are gaining popularity today, which are much more in line with Western images of "masculine" males and "feminine" females, are the same as those in the past, and if they are not, how much of this change is the result of adopting Western standards.

For example, in traditional Thai literature and epics the male heroes were described as having beautiful features, slim bodies, smooth skin, and a soft manner. The leading male stars in *Likay*, the popular musical folk plays, were expected to have this appearance to be described as handsome and desirable by the audience. This same image was identified with the aristocrats as well, while those with dark skin, a muscular build, and a rough manner were generally seen as members of the lower classes.

Another major difference between Thai and Western cultures comes in terms of the lack of social restraints on physical contacts between members of the same sex. Some Western cultures severely restrict allowed forms of public same-sex contact, the result of negative attitudes toward homosexuality that are an outgrowth of Christianity. In Thai society, it is common for members of the same sex, whether having a close relationship or not, to be involved in a great deal of physical contact and touching. It is not uncommon to see two boys or two girls walking down the street holding hands or with arms around each other's shoulders. Often they spend their nights at one another's homes, sharing beds. Kissing a member of the same sex on the cheek in public can be a joking way of expressing affection. The lack of social constraints on physical contact facilitates many of the boys' having their first experiences with sexual excitation with other boys. While in the West this would be considered homosexual activity and would be severely sanctioned as sinful or deviant behavior, there is no associated religious guilt in Thai culture. If these boys go on to have heterosexual contacts with girlfriends or female sex workers while they continue having same-sex contacts, this might be identified by society as bisexual behavior in a Western context, although the Thais might not perceive it in this way at all.

By contrast, in Thai society, the strong social sanctions are reserved for physical and sexual contacts between males and females, not between members of the same sex. It is worth noting that Western influences are starting to break down the barriers proscribing contact between the opposite sexes, while at the same time light sanctions are developing on same-sex physical contacts in public.

Another factor in Thai society that may affect the forms bisexuality may take is strong social pressure toward marriage. Traditionally, Thai males are expected to enter the Buddhist monkhood for a period of time and then to marry upon leaving. In spite of the recent trend toward urbanization, Thailand is still a predominantly agricultural society, with the majority of the people living in rural settings. This creates pressure for individuals to marry for several reasons. There is a strong desire to see the family line continued. In earlier Thai society, the choice of marital partner was often made by the parents. Since the settings are small rural communities, the failure to marry can often lead to gossip among the neighbors. Finally, there are strong socio-economic reasons for marrying because it brings the spouse and children into the family labor pool, providing additional hands to work in the fields. In this environment, even if a man or woman has sexual preferences for members of the same sex, the social pressures will encourage marriage, forcing the individual to look to bisexual contact outside the marital relationship for some of his/her sexual release. This situation and the associated pressures still exist to a lesser degree among the new urban middle-class generation (Anonymous 1990).

ACCOUNTS OF BISEXUALITY

There do exist some accounts of bisexual behavior in Thailand. It is recorded historically, for example, that in the Royal Court, the living quarters of the king and queen where only females were allowed, there was sex between the women. This was a form of situational homosexuality that filled both sexual desires and needs for companionship. There was even a special term to describe sex between women in the court. Later many of these women would leave the court to marry. It is unknown whether they continued same-sex behaviors after this time, but their life experience clearly involved sexual contacts with members of both sexes.

Anecdotal reports indicate the existence of a class of individuals known as *kratuei*. In its original meaning it referred to anyone of either sex who liked to dress up or behave as a member of the opposite sex or liked to have sex with the same sex. These days it has taken on the meaning of a man who likes to dress up or behave as a woman. There are reports (Bunnag 1990a) of *kratuei* men attending parties organized at military bases in Bangkok twenty-five to thirty years ago. The *kratuei* considered these parties to be major events and dressed up for them. The author reports that there would often be competition between the *kratuei* and women at the dances over some of the military men. The military men were aware that the *kratuei* were men, but some still danced with them and dated them. Many of these men had wives, while others were single but would later go on to marry. While men having sex with both women and transvestites was not generally accepted societally, in the context of military-base parties it was not subject to social sanctions.

The existence of linguistic terms can often reveal the presence or social recognition of certain behaviors and norms. In premodern Thailand there were other terms used to describe bisexuality in an indirect fashion. For example, *chob tang song yang,* which translates as "liking both ways," meant that the person, either male or female, liked having sex with both men and women. The term *sua bi* (a fierce thief named Bi) referred to someone who can or did have sex with both men and women, with no clear-cut implication of where the person's true sexual preference lay. These days, with the increasing openness in discussing sexual matters, new terms have entered the language with more specific meanings, for example, "gay" for men who prefer sex with men though they need not have exclusively male partners or announce themselves openly as homosexual; *tut,* a modern substitute for *kratuei,* which became popular after the movie *Tootsie* in which actor Dustin Hoffman dressed up as a woman; and *sao praped song* (the second type of woman) for a man who dresses up as a woman or a transsexual. The term *aab* (hiding) is used to describe men who like to have sex with men but do not want to admit it to themselves or are sensitive and paranoid about their homosexual behavior. Often the term is used for married men who have extramarital sex with other men.

There are also terms to describe women, either single or married, who have sex with women. *Tom* (from the English "tomboy") is used to describe women who appear or would like to appear as men, and *dee* (from the English "lady") is used for those who prefer a feminine appearance. These terms are used without regard to the women's experience with the opposite sex. *Saw* (from the Chinese for "elder sister") is another word used to describe women who come to massage parlors for sex with the masseuses. Based on in-depth interviews, the number of *saw* who are married is higher than the number who are single.

Anecdotal reports in gay magazines frequently describe bisexual situations. One such report (Bunnag 1990b) describes the difficulties of a man who hides his sexual preference for men carefully, even to the point of marrying, and his struggle over whether or not to tell his wife his sexual preference. In the end, he did tell his wife but continued having sex with men while living with his wife and children. Another report (Bunnag 1990c) describes two male bar workers who have bisexual experiences before their orientations later shift toward men.

Modern pornography produced and sold in Thailand sometimes portrays bisexual contacts, usually in the context of trios of one man and two women. Bisexuality in the form of two males and a woman with sex between the men and with the woman is still rare, as it appears to be more acceptable to see homosexuality between women rather than between men. How much of this is due to Western influences is unclear.

MODERN PATTERNS OF BISEXUALITY IN THAILAND

With the above as background, it is time to turn to a discussion of modern patterns of bisexuality. The reader is reminded that this is a description of some of the existing patterns, but that little actual research has been done. It is also worth mentioning that many of the forms of men having sex with men or women with women will rarely lead to any form of self-identification among the Thai as bisexual or homosexual. This is important to remember when analyzing studies that ask questions of self-identification. Because of social restrictions on open discussion of sexual matters, such questions may not give much information about the actual behaviors in which an individual engages. From the point of view of HIV transmission, the behaviors matter more than the self-identification.

The first category is what can be termed early bisexuality. In this form, given the lack of sanctions on same-sex contacts as mentioned above, individuals may experiment with members of the same sex while undergoing integration into the publicly heterosexual pattern that will apply for most of their lives. For many Thai males, part of this integration involves visiting female sex workers. In other cases, some male adolescents at the earliest stages of their sexual lives are seduced or pressured to have sex with older men. Since there is no strong guilt associated with sexual behaviors, it is possible that some people find sexual contacts with both sexes enjoyable and continue regularly or occasionally to practice bisexual contacts later in life. No studies have been done that explore the extent and nature of same-sex contacts during the formative years in Thai adolescents. However, college surveys (Sakondhavat et al. 1988; Chompootaweep et al. 1988) do exist that show that a large number of the male students have visited female sex workers, and that a few of them admit to having had sexual contacts with other men.

The second category of bisexuality consists of those who have a strong preference for members of one sex or the other, but who choose encounters with the nonpreferred sex for either social or economic reasons. An example of the first would be the man described above who prefers sex with men, but who marries for reasons of social conformity. Because of social pressures, he will be required to have sex with his wife and produce offspring, but his true sexual interests are elsewhere. A few of these cases have become publicly known, particularly after a divorce when the wives spread the news. Further evidence comes from bar workers at male bars who have reported that many of their customers are in fact married. Social pressures may also take other forms, e.g., peer-group pressure. An example of this is one young man who prefers homosexual contacts but visits female sex workers as part of social activities with his friends.

Social pressures are not restricted to men. An in-depth interview with a village woman revealed that she was pressured by her parents to get married and have children. During her married life, she still occasionally had sex with her female lover. After she divorced her husband, she lived openly with her female lover who helped to raise her child.

Examples of economic reasons for bisexuality are found in the sexual-service industry itself, which is extensive and well-developed in Thailand. (The existence of the sexual service industry is primarily a response to indigenous demand; however, in many areas it was accelerated by the American presence in the Viet Nam era and has been sustained by the tourist industry.) If one examines men working in male go-go bars, one finds that many of the men describe themselves as heterosexual in preference, often with girlfriends or wives on the side, but commercially engaging in sex with men because it is economically attractive. In one survey conducted by the Thai Red Cross Society among 141 male bar workers in Bangkok (Sittitrai et al. 1989), it was found that 82 percent of the men had taken the job because of unemployment. In the two weeks prior to the interviews, 100 percent had sex with male customers, 23 percent with female customers, 13 percent with noncustomer males, and 50 percent with noncustomer females. It should be stressed that regardless of their actual sexual preferences, many of the male bar workers have long-term partners, some male lovers but the majority girlfriends or wives.

Bangkok has several bars with male workers in which only female customers are allowed. However, in-depth interviews reveal that sometimes transvestites or transsexual men utilize the services of the boys. In addition, some of these boys have male customers, but contacts are made outside of the work setting. Bisexual activities are not confined to only the male bars; there have also been a few reports from the female bar workers and massage parlor girls of married women coming in for sexual services from other women.

Another aspect of this sexual trade is that it is not uncommon to find adolescents in the parks who will engage in sex with men in order to pick up additional money. With little of the guilt or social sanctions associated with these behaviors in Western cultures, it is merely viewed as an additional service that can be done in the pursuit of economic gain. From that point of view, it can be quite lucrative, with an individual earning a great deal of money from customers in a short period of time for something which can be mutually enjoyable. The majority of these men selling sex, both in the bars and outside, do become sexually excited and climax with their customers. As one bar boy put it: "If the customer is good in bed, I enjoy sex with him also." Another one said: "Sex is sex, a turn-on is a turn-on, you get hard and come anyway with male or female, especially when you are still young and virile."

The third category of bisexuality is situational bisexuality, that is bisexuality that arises when there are limited opportunities for contact with members of the opposite sex, for example, in prisons or in military bases. Experiences in prison settings have been reported through magazine columns (Anonymous 1989) and in-depth interviews with released prisoners. The existence of homosexual behaviors can be seen in the development of linguistic terms to describe the sexual acts and the roles played in homosexual contacts in prison. These contacts constitute only a portion of the lifetime sexual experience of the prisoners, the majority of whom are married or will later marry. In-depth interviews with military recruits reveal that having sex with "buddies" was used as a means of sexual release when they could not get out to visit female sex workers or girlfriends.

The next category is what one would class as true bisexuals, i.e., those who actually do enjoy sexual contacts with both sexes and maintain bisexual behavioral patterns throughout their lives. For each individual, the degree of sexual experience with each of the genders may vary, from mostly experience with men and occasionally with women, to the opposite extreme of mostly with women and occasionally with men. We have no accurate way of assessing the size of this population in Thailand and the social restrictions on discussing sexual behavior do not make it easy for individuals to identify themselves as such. However, given permissive Thai attitudes toward sexuality and the ease of locating either male or female sexual contacts through the sexual-service outlets, there is little question that most of these individuals can engage in sex with either gender if they so desire.

There is a final category of bisexual behavior and preference. This is the men who prefer sex with transvestites or transsexuals. Strictly speaking, they should not be classed as homosexual since they prefer to have sex with persons having both male and female features and appearances in the same body. The existence of this form of bisexuality is illustrated by the case of one young man whose love is a transsexual. He says he gets turned on the most by a man who has female genitals as a result of an operation. This form of bisexuality will likely be practiced by only a small number of individuals.

EXISTING DATA ON BISEXUAL CONTACTS

There are no direct studies of bisexuality in Thailand. One study that has asked questions about sexual experience is the Survey of Partner Relations and Risk of HIV Infection, sponsored by the World Health Organization and carried out by the Thai Red Cross Society and Chulalongkorn University. Respondents were asked to characterize their lifetime sexual experience in terms of the gender of their partners as shown in table 1.

The people represented in three middle categories of this table (mostly with women, equally with women and men, and mostly with men) have engaged in sexual activities—defined here as anal, oral, or vaginal, or genital-to-genital intercourse—with both males and females. It should be noted that mutual masturbation, e.g., in the context of early bisexuality,

TABLE 1
Gender of Partners in Sexual Activity

	% Men (n = 983)	% Women (n = 1285)
Only had sex with women	96.5	0.9
Mostly had sex with women, but sometimes with men	2.8	0.1
Had sex equally with women and men	0.2	0.1
Mostly had sex with men, but sometimes with women	0.1	0.2
Only had sex with men	0.3	98.8

would not be captured in these figures. These results show that 3.1 percent of the male interviewees and 0.4 percent of the female interviewees indicated that they had sexual experiences with both sexes. It is expected that these numbers underreport the actual level of such activities. Little difference was seen in these percentages between rural and urban areas.

Another part of this study bearing on questions of bisexuality was a section inquiring about definitions of "having sex." In this section, respondents were asked about which forms of male/female, male/male, and female/female sexual behavior they considered to be "having sex." Table 2 lists the percentages of males and females who thought that each of the behaviors listed constituted "having sex." As can be seen from the table, only 25 percent of the men and 22.5 percent of the women consider oral sex between men as "having sex." This implies that the majority of the males in the fifteen-to-forty-nine age group surveyed might not consider their same-sex orogenital experience as placing them in the bisexual category. In addition, less than half of the men and women consider anal intercourse between males to be "having sex." If this is the case, then interventions that are not explicit in terms of HIV risk behaviors but are targeted at using condoms while "having sex" generally may fail to provide sufficient information for many men practicing anal risk behaviors to identify themselves as being

TABLE 2

Definitions of "Having Sex" (Sexual Intercourse) (n = 2902)

	% Male	% Female
Man caressing/kissing a woman	19.4	24.9
Man caressing/kissing a man	6.8	7.4
Woman caressing/kissing a woman	7.4	7.0
Placing penis in vagina	98.3	98.3
Male placing penis in male anus	48.7	44.2
Male/female orogenital	33.6	33.8
Male/male orogenital	25.0	22.5

TABLE 3
Categorization of Risk Behaviors Reported in
Thailand as of October 31, 1990

	AIDS		ARC*		HIV+	
		%		%		%
Sexual Transmission	53	(76.8)	110	(55.0)	6230	(26.8)
Male homosexual	18	(26.1)	18	(9.0)	76	(0.3)
Male bisexual	9	(13.0)	8	(4.0)	103	(0.4)
Male heterosexual	21	(30.4)	60	(30.0)	2279	(9.8)
Female heterosexual	5	(7.2)	24	(12.0)	3772	(16.2)
IVDUs	8	(11.6)	75	(37.5)	14808	(63.6)
Male	8	(11.6)	73	(36.5)	14236	(61.2)
Female	0	(0.0)	2	(1.0)	572	(2.5)
Blood Transfusion	2	(2.9)	4	(2.0)	31	(0.1)
Male	1	(1.4)	3	(1.5)	19	(0.1)
Female	1	(1.4)	1	(0.5)	12	(0.1)
Vertical Transmission	6	(8.7)	1	(0.5)	0	(0.0)
Male	2	(2.9)	1	(0.5)	0	(0.0)
Female	4	(5.8)	0	(0.0)	0	(0.0)
Unidentified	9	(0.0)	10	(5.0)	2210	(9.5)
Male	0	(0.0)	8	(4.0)	2067	(8.9)
Female	0	(0.0)	2	(1.0)	143	(0.6)
GRAND TOTALS	69	(100.0)	200	(100.0)	23279	(100.0)
Alive (in country)	17	(24.6)	170	(85.0)	23076	(99.1)

Source: Division of AIDS (1990)

at risk. The results of this table further imply that self-identification or societal identification as bisexual may not always occur even in the presence of HIV risk behaviors with both sexes. It is worth noting that there is little difference in opinion between the male and female groups interviewed here.

---

*AIDS-Related Complex (Ed.)

BISEXUALITY AND HIV IN THAILAND

The human immunodeficiency virus (HIV) has made significant inroads in Thailand. Seroprevalence surveys done nationwide show high seroprevalence in intravenous drug users (IVDUs) (30 percent to 40 percent in Bangkok), female sex workers (9.5 percent median, 0 percent to 67 percent range depending on geographic location), and males attending STD clinics (2.5 percent median, 0 percent to 24 percent range) (Division of Epidemiology 1990). Another survey conducted in several provinces shows that HIV seroprevalence among men who come for military recruiting is approximately 10 percent. Interestingly, male sex workers in Thailand generally show lower rates of seroprevalence than the females, and gay men also appear to have comparatively low seroprevalence rates. These differences between the male and female sex workers may be a result of differences in numbers of customers serviced in a night, practice of safer sex in gay encounters, or differing prevalences of other STDs that enhance HIV transmission.

One indicator of the impact of bisexuality on AIDS/HIV is to examine the risk categories reported by individuals presenting with AIDS, ARC, or HIV positivity. These numbers for Thailand as of October 1990 are reproduced in table 3 from the AIDS Newsletter of November 1990 (Division of AIDS 1990).

As can be seen from the table, those reporting male bisexuality as a risk factor constituted 13 percent of the AIDS cases, 4 percent of the ARC cases, and only 0.4 percent of reported HIV positivity. There has been no reporting of female bisexuality as a risk factor. In many societies bisexuals are perceived as a "bridge" population that may allow HIV infection to move from a highly infected subpopulation to a less easily infected population. An example of this is the way bisexual men in large cities in the United States are often viewed as unidirectionally transmitting HIV between heavily infected gay communities and "lower-risk" heterosexual communities.

In Thailand the situation appears to be much more complicated. Given the high levels of HIV infection in various subpopulations, the high prevalences of other HIV-transmission enhancing STDs, especially in the lower income sex workers, and the general permissiveness of Thai society, it is possible that there may be an intricate pattern of bidirectional flow of HIV between various segments of the population, including IVDUs, heterosexual males, sex workers, gay men, and wives/partners of each of these groups. In this complex network of contacts,

FIGURE 1
Possible Bisexual Networks of HIV Transmission in Thailand

(a)

Network Involving Bisexual Male Bar Workers

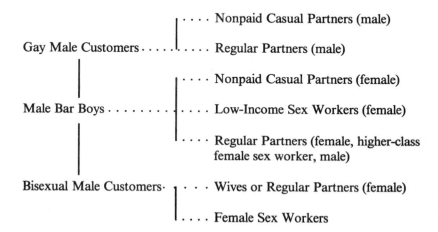

(b)

Network Involving Situational Bisexuality in Prisons with IVDUs

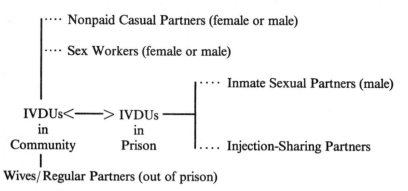

FIGURE 1 (contd.)

(c)

Early Bisexuality

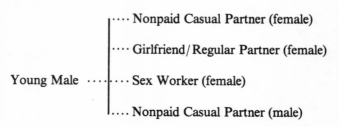

bisexuals may play several key roles. Figure 1 illustrates some of the potentially important bisexual networks of HIV transmission in Thai society, as depicted from the results of surveys and qualitative studies. Please note that these are not intended to be comprehensive or complete, but to illustrate the level of complexity that may arise in analyzing the situation in Thailand. Note further that in the current Thai context, many of the avenues shown here may as easily support HIV transmission from female to male as from male to female. For reference, estimated sizes of some of the more important subpopulations are male sex workers, 5000–8000; female sex workers, 150,000–200,000; and IVDUs approximately 200,000. Bear in mind that none of these is a static population; there are people entering and leaving each of them constantly at rates that maintain them at approximately this size. This is particularly true of the sex workers who have a very high turnover rate and mobility.

At this point, given the infection rates in the different subpopulations, the major risk factors in Thailand are intravenous drug usage and heterosexual intercourse with sex workers and customers of sex workers. This may create a novel situation in which bisexuality may serve as a bridge into gay populations with lower infection rates from higher seroprevalence heterosexual populations (fig. 1a). Many of the male sex workers who have sexual preference for females visit female sex workers on their own time. While gay men and male sex workers in Thailand are well educated on issues of HIV transmission, it is possible in some cases that the perception of risk may extend only or primarily to contacts with gay men. The male sex workers may then feel less risk (or no risk) in engaging in unprotected intercourse with female sex workers and thus increase their chance of heterosexual infection. In one northern

Thai province, it was found that the HIV seroprevalence among male bar workers rose from 2 percent in December 1989 to 18 percent in June 1990. Epidemiological and behavioral data show that the HIV-infected bar boys had unprotected sex with female sex workers among whom the seroprevalence rates were very high. Once infected, their failure to abide by safer-sex rules may result in infection of their male customers.

Another possible route of bisexual infection is between the male sex worker and his regular female partner (girlfriend or wife). If the worker is pressured into unsafe sex at work, he may become infected homosexually. Numerous interviews with the sex workers have shown that many of them do not use any form of protection in their opposite-sex relationships. Given higher male-to-female transmission rates, it becomes quite possible they may infect their female partners. This may also extend to the women they marry after they have left the sexual-service industry and thus possibly to their children.

Bisexuality in prison contexts (fig. 1b) may lead to high rates of HIV transmission. Current figures show that while 40 percent of the people going into prison are HIV-infected, 55 percent of those tested at exit time are. Whether this is transmission occurring through situational homosexuality, needle sharing in the prisons, or both is unclear, but the potential for spread to sexual or needle-sharing partners after release is obvious. In-depth interviews with male IVDUs in a Bangkok slum and in a northern province reveal that they have had sexual experience with both males and females. There is one case of a bisexual male who met his IVDU transvestite lover in prison. The two continued to be lovers for two years after their release, while the bisexual man secretly had sex with other women in the slum community (Sittitrai et al. 1990).

It is also unclear what role early bisexuality (fig. 1c) or experimentation with both sexes may play in HIV spread. Since the sexual behaviors in this stage have not been characterized but do often involve visiting sex workers with neither the awareness nor the motivation to practice safer sex, it is quite possible that infection through heterosexual contact may then result in infection of other males through homosexual contacts or vice versa. There is also the potential for spread to both casual and regular female partners. Clearly, further research on this topic is in order.

FUTURE RESEARCH NEEDS

To understand the developing patterns of HIV transmission in Thailand and develop effective interventions, it is important to consider the place and role of Thai bisexuality. However, given how poorly it is characterized at present, there is a strong need for additional work. The first piece of research suggested is a series of mini-surveys and in-depth qualitative studies for confirmation of the patterns of bisexuality that have been proposed here. Based on observations, scattered data, and anecdotal evidence, this chapter has presented one possible view of Thai bisexuality that is by no means conclusive.

The prevalence of the various forms of bisexual behavior must be determined and the settings in which they occur characterized, particularly among Thai husbands and the sex worker population. Given the complexity of the bisexual networks outlined above, a mapping study of the social and sexual networks of bisexuals must be undertaken if the relationship between HIV spread and bisexuality in Thai society is to be understood. It is important to learn how partners are selected, the frequency with which bisexuals interact with others, how much use is made of sex worker outlets, and what the types of sexual risk behavior are practiced with each of the genders or categories of partners.

In designing interventions to reach Thai bisexuals, it will be necessary to know whether they self-identify as bisexual, how they perceive themselves, and how society perceives them. Do they consider themselves part of a larger bisexual community? If so, what form does this community take, who are its opinion leaders, and what are the communication networks? What are the current and future trends of public attitudes toward bisexuality: positive, negative, or neutral? How might these attitudes help or hinder attempts to reach this group?

Issues of sexual perception must also be examined more closely. As the Survey of Partner Relations has indicated, for some portion of the population not all sexual activities in a bisexual context are considered to be "having sex." If interventions are not quite explicit in explaining possible means of HIV transmission, these perceptions may result in prevention messages being misunderstood or misinterpreted.

Information on the AIDS/HIV knowledge, attitudes, and practices of Thai bisexuals must be gathered with particular attention to feelings of relative risk of different sexual behaviors. As mentioned above, individuals engaging in bisexual behaviors may have different patterns of condom use depending on the gender of their partner or their relationship to that partner. This calls for caution and care in developing interventions; for example, to give the impression that anal sex is much riskier than vaginal sex may lead to continued heterosexual high-risk behaviors on the part of individuals who make poor personal risk assessments. In the Thai context with high rates of transmission between female sex workers and their customers, misperceptions of this type may have lethal consequences.

Instead, the emphasis in all interventions must be on the constant practice of safer sex and reduction of other risk behaviors. Because of the complexity of bisexual behaviors in Thailand, it may not be possible to identify a distinct "target group" for intervention, implying that only a minority of individuals with bisexual behaviors may be reachable through bisexual contact networks. If this is the case, then most of these individuals will have to be reached as part of the general population, by education about risk behaviors.

The patterns of HIV transmission in Thailand may be among the most complex in the world. Characterizing these patterns so as to target the most effective interventions will require a solid understanding of sexuality in all of its forms in Thailand, especially bisexuality. Given the urgency of the needs and the seriousness of the situation, small-scale, rapid, in-depth, intervention-geared research deserves the priority. With the pivotal role that bisexuality may play, this research cannot begin too soon.

10

Patterns of Bisexuality in Indonesia

Dédé Oetomo

INTRODUCTION

This is a preliminary attempt to map patterns of bisexuality in present-day Indonesia. It is necessarily preliminary in nature because systematic research on this phenomenon has so far simply not been carried out. As such, what is described here is based on:

1. participant observation in different sections of Indonesian society, specifically, homosexual and transvestite/transsexual communities; and

2. experience in conducting peer-counseling, either directly or by correspondence, with members of the aforementioned communities and individuals.

Indonesia is an archipelagic republic with a population of 180 million inhabitants. When talking about it, especially as it concerns human behavior, one must recognize its diversity. There are 300 different ethnic groups; a few, like the Javanese, consist of as many as 80 million people, but many small population groups are made up of as few as 100 people. Most ethnic groups have been in the area for thousands of years, but there are also ethnic Chinese, Arabs, and Indians. All major religions are found, with Islam being by far the dominant one. About 20 percent of the population is urban, while 80 percent is rural. This also means in most cases a discrepancy in literacy and education (i.e., more in urban areas), income and wealth (also higher in urban areas), and modernization/Westernization (urban centers being more modernized/Westernized).

So it is with this backdrop of diversity that the following description is laid out. The discussion is limited to the area administratively designated as the Republic of Indonesia. The limitation is obviously artificial, but it is assumed that after more than forty years of independence, enough coherence can be found in (especially modern) Indonesian society to warrant treating the country as a single social unit.

SEXUAL CATEGORIES IN INDONESIAN SOCIETY

Before discussing bisexuality itself, it is important to survey briefly the sexual categories into which Indonesian society assigns its members.

Most Indonesians group people into three genders, namely, male (*laki-laki*), female (*perempuan*) and an in-between, third gender called *banci, wadam,* or *waria* (throughout this article, we shall use the last term, which is preferred by these people themselves in formal usage). Although on the surface it seems that only males and females matter in Indonesian society in connection with institutions like marriage and the family, and regular heterosexuality is the dominant norm, Indonesians do refer to certain types of people as *waria.* These are either (1) people who appear androgynous or behave androgynously, or (2) biological males who cross-dress, adopt the behavior and societal roles of females, identify themselves as *waria,* and socialize regularly with fellow *warias* in definable communities. Thus, whereas the first definition of *waria* refers to a description of an androgynous gender behavior, the second definition refers to a socially constructed identity. A rather cumbersome translation of *waria* as a certain type of person is thus "transvestite or transsexual male homosexual." What is significant and should be mentioned here is that non-cross-dressing and gender-conforming male homosexuals are considered *warias* by all but a very few modern, educated, Western-oriented Indonesians. It should also be noted that female homosexuals (*lesbis*) are rarely discussed by the general public in terms of the *waria* identity, although sometimes their behavior may be described as *waria*-like.

Within the communities of *warias,* gays, and lesbians, the social categories are different. *Lesbis* are an easily separable category and are never mixed up with the other two. While most of the general public lump together *warias* and male homosexuals, in the communities themselves there is an almost watertight distinction between *warias* on the one hand and *homos* or gays on the other. While some *homos* may at one time or another cross-dress or even adopt a *waria* identity in a different locale (e.g., in a different town) and while many of them behave androgynously, the greater majority of them see themselves as significantly different from *warias*. In Indonesia's urban centers, this is often manifested in separate communities, separate hang-outs, and so forth. There may even be animosity between the two groups mainly because many *warias* are sex workers while some *homos* pay for sex. Often the *warias* see that men who are their potential clients may prefer *homos* because instead of paying for sex, they are paid for it. A few preliminary surveys also show that *warias* tend to be of working-class background, while *homos* are members of the middle class or at least aspire to be so (Oetomo 1988: 37–38).

It should be mentioned that except for categories in various traditional cultures, *warias, homos,* and *lesbis* are modern categories imported from the West. This does not imply that homosexual behavior is not known in traditional, non-Westernized Indonesian cultures (for general surveys, see Kroef 1954; Herdt 1984; Oetomo 1988). It just means that except for a few cases of institutionalized homosexuality known to occur, we are not sure if such traditional manifestations elsewhere have not been eradicated by the advent of modernization (e.g., in the form of conversion to Christianity). Since in-depth research has not been conducted, we cannot be fully sure if they continue to exist. In addition, it is important to point out that homosexual behavior is never perceived as a special category of sexual behavior by traditional Indonesian cultures; in other words, where it is recognized, it is always associated with some culturally well-integrated institution. Moreover, it is necessary to realize that homosexual behavior is very rarely carried out mutually exclusive to heterosexual behavior, although in some cultures during certain culturally significant periods only one type of behavior (homosexual or heterosexual) is prescribed.

Modern Indonesians tolerate their *waria* compatriots quite well on a societal level, but families often have a hard time, at least initially, accepting that one of their members is a *waria*. Except among a small group of highly educated people, the attitude toward *homos* and *lesbis* on an intellectual, cognitive level is mostly one of nonacceptance of a deviant behavior often considered immoral and sinful. However, in terms of actual behavior vis-à-vis homosexual men and women one actually knows or encounters, the attitude is one of silent tolerance and of "live and let live."

WHO HAS SEX WITH WHOM, AND HOW?

To understand patterns of bisexuality in Indonesia, one must take into account the way *warias, homos,* and *lesbis* regard the people with whom they have sex.

Sex Between and With *Warias*

Warias very rarely have sex with each other, although from interviews in the field such intercourse does happen from time to time. The same is true of sex between a *waria* and a *homo.* In fact, once it is established that a potential male partner is actually a *homo,* most *warias* refuse to continue their seduction. Different sexual techniques are used: oral, anal, interfemoral,* frottage,† and (mutual) masturbation. There is no definable pattern as to who should be the inserter and who the insertee.

In most cases *warias* have sex with men whom they identify as *laki-laki* (males). Many find their *waria* partners in publicly known hang-outs ("street beats," parks, and amusement centers). Encounters can also happen in beauty parlors, where many *warias* work as hairdressers or beauticians, and in the context of traditional performances where female roles are played by *warias.* Since most *warias* live openly in regular neighborhoods, it is conceivable that encounters also take place in such contexts. Well-to-do *warias* often pay male prostitutes to have sex with them.

Men who have sex with *warias* are not considered homosexual by the general public, *warias,* or by themselves. Although one might guess that sex with *warias* is considered part of adolescent experimentation, one also finds adult, married men having sex with *warias* on a regular basis. Despite the fact that female prostitution is widely available in most Indonesian urban centers (and even in some rural areas), these men persist in having sex with *warias.* This probably signifies that they do prefer sex with *warias* to sex with women. There are two generally

*Between the thighs (Ed.)
†A rubbing movement, as in massage (Ed.)

expressed rationalizations for this: (1) sex with *warias* does not pose the risk of pregnancy and hence the possibility of being forced to marry; and (2) sex with *warias* is safe from the risk of contracting sexually transmitted diseases (STDs). Different sexual techniques are used in these encounters. What is interesting and significant is the fact that in some cases the "men" do become the insertee in both anal and oral sex. It is also worth mentioning that a very few of these men eventually adopt androgynous behavior, cross-dress, and become *warias* themselves.

It might be useful to point out that sex within marriage is considered more procreational than recreational. In fact, it is safe to say that in Indonesian society marriage is almost a duty one has to perform for society, religion, and so forth, but almost invariably not something based on romantic love and passion as such. Interviews with women indicate that most of them perceive sex in the very limited scope of marriage and as something almost abhorrent. A woman showing that she enjoys sex risks being equated with a prostitute.

A very few *warias* are heterosexually married. Many of their wives do not know of their husbands' other lifestyle, but a very small number do.

Sex Between and With *Homos*

Homos are for all intents and purposes similar to modern gay men in the West. Many gay men are willing to have sex with men who identify themselves as gay, but others prefer *laki-laki* (males), i.e., men who in their own view are not gay. These gay men immediately lose interest once they know that the man they desire has ever performed oral sex on or been anally penetrated by another man. In fact, they are very proud if their partner is a heterosexually married man, since that proves that he is a "real" man. Obviously this is all in the gay men's perception; oftentimes, as long as a gay man does not know that his partner also identifies himself as gay, he considers him a "true" man. From observation in the field, it is almost safe to conclude that many Indonesian men who do not otherwise identify themselves as gay are willing to experiment with homosexuality. Encounters can take place in just about any imaginable locale.

Male sex workers are available in many major urban centers, whether in organized brothels or in publicly known gay hang-outs (parks, "street beats," shopping malls, hotel lobbies, amusement parks, swimming pools, and gyms). Some of these are homosexually inclined, but others are not. Some also have sex with women and *warias*. In fact, one suspects that to many of the so-called *laki-laki, warias,* and *homos* are all in the same category.

As in the case of sex between and with *warias,* once gay men have sex with each other or with *laki-laki,* different sexual techniques may be used, depending on the couple's agreement. Group sex is quite common. It is surprising how many *laki-laki* are willing to engage in any sexual technique in any capacity. One suspects that most Indonesian men do not have sexual hang-ups and are thus easily persuaded to engage in new sexual experiences. There is reason to suspect that this is even easier when the seduction comes from a foreigner (especially Caucasian) or a member of the immigrant communities (Chinese, Arab, or Indian).

In the past two years or so, awareness of safe sexual techniques has increased among gay men, although one cannot be sure whether they actually refrain from engaging in such high-risk behavior.

The pressure from family and society for gay men to get married and set up a family is quite strong and persistent. As a result, many gay men are married once they are in their late twenties or early thirties at the latest. This does not mean that they necessarily stop their homosexual encounters; some do so when traveling, and others lead a double life, which is feasible especially in the anonymity of big cities.

Public knowledge indicates that situational homosexual behavior takes place in dormitories, barracks, and prisons, although we do not know to what extent. Better knowledge is available about institutionalized homosexuality (the technique used is mostly interfemoral intercourse) in orthodox Islamic boarding schools (*pondhok pesantrèn*) in Central and East Java and Madura (called *mairilan* in Javanese or *laq-dalaq* in Madurese), and perhaps also elsewhere (West Java and West Sumatra) where such education exists. This is considered part of the educational process; most of the students stop engaging in homosexual behavior once they leave school. They then get married; a very few continue the relationship with their former lover/fellow student.

Another type of institutionalized homosexuality is prevalent between adult men who search for supernatural prowess (*waroks*) and male youths (*gemblaks*) in the Ponorogo area in western East Java province. Some *waroks* have been married, sometimes to more than one woman. However, at a certain stage in their life, once they feel economically and politically established, they decide, in the course of searching for prowess, to abstain from heterosexual intercourse and enter into a relationship with one or more *gemblaks,* depending on how much they can pay the youths' respective families. The *gemblaks* eventually get married, and a very few go on to become *waroks* themselves.

One might find other such institutionalizations of homosexual behavior in other Indonesian cultures, but for that one must still wait for detailed ethnographies.

Sex Between and With *Lesbis*

Lesbis (for all intents and purposes similar to lesbians in the West) are the least-known population group in Indonesian society. From observation one knows that lesbian couples exist in many parts of Indonesia. There are also certain hang-outs (pubs, restaurants) frequented by lesbians, but such contacts are necessarily limited, given the limitations on going out alone or even in groups, especially at night, that women face in Indonesian society. There have been reports that some lesbians hang out at prostitution complexes and buy sex there, and that a small number of female sex workers are predominantly homosexual. Different sexual techniques are used, including (mutual) masturbation (with or without tools) and frottage.

Since the pressure to get married and set up a family is even stronger on women, most lesbians are, have been, or will be married. However, reports indicate that situational female homosexuality exists in dormitories, prisons, barracks, and other such institutions.

CONCLUSION

Despite the "normal," heterosexual façade that Indonesian society seems to project, there is a great deal of sexual diversity. It is even safe to conclude that one way or the other, many Indonesian males are bisexual, although such a category is not commonly employed outside of academic or journalistic circles.

The dearth of research on bisexuality, or indeed sexuality in general, in Indonesian society means that much research needs to be done before an accurate picture of the phenomenon can be presented. The above exposition is meant to be a preliminary mapping of patterns of bisexuality.

Useful research should be conducted on certain target groups, such as men who have sex with *warias* and *homos,* in terms of their complete sexual behavior. Other target groups may be married gay men as well as married lesbians. In connection with research on the spread of HIV/

AIDS, one must emphasize the need for research on people who the general public assumes are "normal" men but who in actual fact have sex with *warias* and *homos*. Since many of these men are engaged in high-risk behavior and also have sex with women (often concurrently), they should receive top priority in research on bisexuality in connection with the spread of HIV/AIDS.

11

Male Bisexuality in Australia

Michael W. Ross

There has been little published work on bisexuality in Australia, as most research has concentrated on homosexuality and included, but not differentiated, bisexuality. Ross (1983) looked in some detail at one category of bisexual men, men who had married but had sexual contact with other men. He found that for most of his respondents, there was not a conflict between homosexual and heterosexual contacts, although a small proportion had married in order to "remove" their homosexual desires. Regardless of whether the respondents had discovered their homosexual interests before or after marriage, the study demonstrated that there was no necessary incompatability between a heterosexual marriage and homosexual desires, and that most men in such a situation managed to maintain both homosexual and married contacts, even though the majority described themselves as predominantly homosexual in orientation. Comparing Australia with other Western societies, Ross (1983) also found that homosexual men were more likely to have married in those societies that were more antihomosexual and sex-role rigid. In such societies, these homosexual men who had married were likely to fear a more negative societal and personal response to their sexual orientation than those who had not married.

The prevalence of bisexual behavior in Australia can be estimated from several sources. Ross, Freedman, and Brew (1989) studied 173 men recruited from gay bars, discos, bathhouses, and cruising areas. Their sexual contacts in the past two months were as follows: 29 (16.8 percent) had had no sexual contacts; 122 (70.5 percent) had had only male contacts. Eleven (6.4 percent) had had only female contacts, and a further 11 had had both male and female sexual contacts. Given that the data were collected from respondents who all identified as gay, these data from homosexual men suggest that in this urban sample from a city of one million inhabitants, 12.8 percent were behaviorally bisexual (a two-month period prevalence). While it is difficult to compare this with overseas data, which is usually based on whether respondents had *ever* had sex with a female (and hence subject to the bias that it includes what may be "experimental" rather than habitual sexual contact), Saghir and Robins (1978) found that 48 percent of their male homosexual sample had had sex with a woman.

From a *general population* perspective, Ross (1988a,b) reported on a large (over 2,600) random sample of people over sixteen years of age in all states and territories of Australia. The sample was asked about their sexual behavior in the past year, and while over 60 percent returned the HIV risk behavior questionnaire left with them at the conclusion of the interview, the data could be biased by incomplete return rate.

Respondents were asked to indicate whether they had ever had sex with a male or with a female, and if in the affirmative, whether it occurred in the past year. Data indicated that the distribution of homosexual contact in men by marital status was not statistically significant, suggesting that the rates of homosexual contact in married and previously married men were not significantly different from single men. Specifically, 4.2 percent of married men reported that they had had sex with another man in the past year (compared with 9.8 percent of single men and 6.4 percent of previously married men). These data, which indicate that one in 24 married men will have sexual contact with another man, suggest that there is a small but significant group of bisexual men in the Australian community.

When one examines the overall data from this study, the proportion of men who have had sex with both men and women in their lifetime is 6.1 percent; however, when one examines the proportion who report having sex with both males *and* females in the past year, it approaches 1 percent. It would thus appear that the number who are behaviorally (or concurrently) bisexual in any given year may be much lower in this population than those who have had bisexual experience. However, these data are based on a 61 percent response rate for those sampled, and an unknown no-contact or refusal rate, and must be viewed with caution given these methodological problems.

Having sex with both males and females, however, does not necessarily equate with risk of HIV transmission. The nature of the sexual contact may have been "safe" in that condoms were used for penetrative acts, or safe in the sense that the acts did not involve penetration. There is little data that would cast any light on this question in Australia. One study that is of considerable use, however, is a study by Bennett, Chapman, and Bray (1989a) on 114 men who engaged in sexual activity with other men on "beats" (public toilets, parks, or isolated spots where men meet for homosexual encounters). Bennett et al. found that of their sample, 12 percent of those who were having sex with other men on "beats" were married or in de facto relationships with women. Thirty-nine percent of "beat" users described themselves as bisexual and an additional 9 percent as heterosexual, and of the total sample of "beat" users, 83 percent had had contact with women.

Bennett, Chapman, and Bray (1989b) interviewed 54 bisexual men who had reported sexual experiences with both men and women in the past six months and found that 46 percent were engaging in unsafe sexual practices with at least one man and one woman. Their data, while again subject to caveats about unrepresentativeness, do suggest that bisexual men may be at greater risk of engaging in unsafe sexual behaviors than those men who engage in sex solely with other men. Given the fact that a substantial number of men would not speak with interviewers in this study, and that they may have been those more concerned about their behavior and less likely to admit to their behavior, the findings of Bennett et al. (1989a,b) may represent underestimates of risk.

The data on bisexuality in men in Australia, with particular reference to risks of HIV transmission, suggest that there is a small but significant number of men who have sex with both men and women. Those who do not define themselves as predominantly homosexual and use "beats" appear to engage in behaviors that may sexually transmit HIV to a substantial degree, and thus specific research and educational campaigns aimed at this section of the community are both warranted and urgent. However, there is no strong evidence to suggest that bisexuality in men in Australia is in any way different in prevalence and pattern to bisexuality in other Western societies.

12

Bisexuality in New Zealand*

Jane Chetwynd

INTRODUCTION

In common with many other countries, New Zealand has relatively little research information on bisexuals. In fact, until recently, bisexuality has hardly been acknowledged as a legitimate sexual orientation, let alone a subject for legitimate research. Bisexuals have been marginalized in New Zealand society as they have in many others. They have been subject to both heterosexism and homosexism and excluded from both the straight and gay communities (Came 1988).

This marginalization is reflected in the way that research on bisexuals has been reported. Studies on populations that include bisexual men invariably present aggregated findings for "homosexuals" (e.g., Rosser 1988a). Studies of lesbian women rarely mention bisexuality even when the topic is a related one such as motherhood (e.g., Knight 1983). The result is that research information on bisexuals is inaccessible and underanalyzed. A recent bibliography of all published and unpublished literature on New Zealand sexuality had no entries under the heading of bisexuality and the topic was not listed in the subject index (Hill and Crothers 1988).

---

*My thanks to Kay Gubbins of the Wellington Bisexual Women's Group, Lois Nunn of the New Zealand AIDS Foundation Library, and the staff of the Canterbury Medical Library.

Bisexuality has not only been hidden from view and marginalized, but it has also been medicalized. So, for example, a series of reports on married homosexuals took the perspective that these men were maladjusted (Ross 1978, 1982, 1983). Interestingly, this maladjustment was not seen to be because of their homosexuality, as it might have been twenty years ago, but rather the implicit assumption was that their bisexuality was the cause of their pathology.

Recent events have seen a change in attitudes to, and concern about, bisexuality in New Zealand. The decriminalization of homosexuality in 1986 gave legitimacy and legality to bisexual men. Of greater impact was the onset of the HIV epidemic, which has resulted in considerable research interest in bisexuals as a group in their own right. This greater interest, however, has tended to be motivated by a concern about the likelihood of spread of the epidemic to the majority heterosexual population, rather than by any particular concern for the health of bisexuals themselves.

A confounding problem in describing research findings concerning bisexuality is that of definition. In many studies bisexuality is defined in terms of genital sexual activity. In others it is seen as a function of sexual orientation or sexual identification. An illustration of the impact of differing definitions is provided by a recent study of homosexual men in Auckland (Rosser 1988b). On the basis of their sexual experience in the previous three years, 25 percent of the sample could be defined as bisexuals, whereas in terms of their nominated sexual identity, 35 percent were so defined.

Bisexuals themselves often prefer a broader definition. For example, the Wellington Bisexual Women's Group support the following definition: "Bisexuals are people who experience the desire for emotional, sensual and/or sexual relationships with people of both sexes, although not necessarily to an equal extent or at the same time" (London Bisexual Collective 1988).

Where possible in this chapter the definition that has been used in a particular study will be identified when findings are discussed.

Because of the recent upsurge of interest in bisexuality there are now some relevant research studies underway in New Zealand, although many of them are ongoing and not yet published. This chapter will cover what we know about the incidence of bisexuality in New Zealand and the sociodemographic characteristics of bisexuals; their sexual practices including condom usage; the context of sexual contacts; changes in sexual practices in response to HIV and motivations for these changes;

health and welfare of bisexuals; and, in the final section, research needs in this area.

INCIDENCE AND DEMOGRAPHY

Incidence

We have very little information on which to base estimates of the incidence of bisexuality in New Zealand. In 1987 a national sample of New Zealanders was surveyed about its knowledge, attitudes, beliefs, and practices concerning AIDS (Chetwynd 1987). An anonymous, self-completed section of the questionnaire concerned self-descriptions of sexual identity/ practices. The results showed that 1.4 percent of the sample described themselves as bisexual in terms of sexual practice. When the study was repeated in 1989 the proportion was 0.8 percent (Department of Health 1989). A recent study of attendees at a Family Planning Clinic showed a similar proportion (1.3 percent) describing themselves as bisexual (Branden 1990–).

It can be argued that quantitative survey approaches are not likely to yield honest results about sexual practices or feelings, and that these findings are likely to be underestimates as a consequence. However, their value lies in providing a lowest bound to the estimate.

Race

Maori people make up 9 percent of the New Zealand population, but there is no information on bisexuality or homosexuality among them. Early suggestions that there were no "sexual deviants" among the Maoris before the European settlement (Gluckman 1974) have now been refuted as a reflection of the reporting practices and narrowness of the missionaries rather than the reality of Maori life (MacFarlane 1984). On the contrary, there is evidence of larger numbers of transsexuals among Maoris than among the European population (MacFarlane 1984; Chetwynd and Hughes 1990) and this has led to the suggestion that the Maoris may allow greater variation of sexual expression. This in turn may be because of the stronger sense of kinship among the Maoris than among the European population (MacFarlane 1984).

Age and Class

There are no studies giving information about age or class characteristics of bisexual people. Studies of adolescent sexuality have tended to focus only on heterosexual practices and related issues (e.g., Lewis 1987), or have described sexual practices in such broad terms that the sexual orientation of the respondents has not been made clear (e.g., Lord 1980).

Incidence of HIV/AIDS

Even in the crucial area of HIV/AIDS statistics we do not know rates of infection among bisexual people. Information on risk behavior is collected for all reported cases of AIDS, but the figures for bisexual and homosexual men are combined. This means that incidence in the two groups cannot be separated out. To date there have been 175 reported cases of people with AIDS in New Zealand, and 85 percent of these have been among homosexual or bisexual men (University of Otago, Dunedin 1990). There have been none reported among bisexual women.

SEXUAL PRACTICES

A good source of information on bisexuality in New Zealand is the AIDS Foundation that collected data during its counseling of people requesting HIV testing. This testing is carried out completely anonymously, and confidentiality is assured because only false names are used in the clinics (Chetwynd 1989). During the counseling session extensive information about sexual identity, practices, and health is collected. Analysis of the results is ongoing, but preliminary findings are available for the most recent 815 people attending the Burnett Clinic in Auckland (Chetwynd and Hughes 1990). Of these people 13 percent described their sexual orientation as bisexual. There were 80 men and 25 women. Descriptions of their sexual practices in an average month showed that oral sex was the most commonly reported practice by men, being cited by 85 percent of the sample. Among women, 68 percent reported participation in oral sex. Vaginal intercourse was reported by 71 percent of men and 80 percent of women, receptive anal intercourse by 60 percent of men and 40 percent of women, and active anal intercourse by 64 percent of men.

Condom usage during anal intercourse was also described. Among the men, 38 percent reported using condoms with casual partners and 21 percent with regular partners. Just over half the men (54 percent) reported generally positive feelings about the use of condoms; however, breakages were reported by 10 percent. None of the bisexual women reported the use of condoms in anal intercourse, but 52 percent of them reported positive feelings about condom use in general.

CONTEXT OF SEXUAL CONTACTS

The study described above also included information on the context in which sexual contacts were made, but this was only for the men. Pubs and clubs were the most common contact point reported by 35 percent of the men, and the same proportion made contact through friends or other social events. Saunas were reported as a contact place by 28 percent, public toilets by 24 percent, beaches by 21 percent, and parks by 18 percent. Only small proportions reported using brothels, massage parlors, or other forms of prostitution. These findings were very similar for the gay men in the sample.

CHANGES IN RESPONSE TO HIV

There is some evidence that gay and bisexual men in New Zealand have changed their sexual practices in response to the emergence of HIV (Rosser 1988b; Parkinson and Hughes 1987; Marshall 1990). Unfortunately, the studies to date have combined responses from both groups so that no separate findings on bisexual men are available. However, one study looking at motivations for sexual change has provided some insights into changes among bisexual men (Horne, Chetwynd, and Kelleher 1989). This study found that those bisexual men practicing unsafe sex were generally uncomfortable with their sexuality and lacked a sense of sexual identification. This was in contrast to some of the gay men who had a strong sexual identity and had made changes toward safer sex. This finding can be interpreted as further evidence of the impact of marginality on bisexuals. Another finding from the study was that among the bisexual men who had changed to safer sex, several of them had done so to protect their wives from infection.

HEALTH AND WELFARE OF BISEXUALS

The study of people attending the AIDS Foundation Clinics also provided extensive information on the health levels and health practices of the bisexuals in that sample (MacFarlane 1984). Full details cannot be given here, but some of the key findings will be presented. Medical histories of sexually transmitted diseases showed that among bisexual women, 28 percent reported genital herpes; 24 percent, genital warts; 16 percent, gonorrhea; and 12 percent, chlamydia. These rates were considerably higher than those among the lesbians in the sample and somewhat higher than the heterosexual women.

Bisexual men reported rates similar to the gay men. For example, 11 percent reported genital herpes; 10 percent, genital warts; 6 percent, anal warts; 16 percent, nonspecific urethritis; and 21 percent, gonorrhea. In terms of emotional health, 20 percent of the bisexual men and 8 percent of the women presented with symptoms of depression, while similar numbers presented with anxiety feelings. Sexual abuse in childhood was reported by 26 percent of the men and 8 percent of the women. Stresses within their current relationships were reported by 40 percent of the men and 60 percent of the women.

Information on drug use was also obtained. Alcohol was the most common drug used by 88 percent of the bisexuals, a similar proportion to that of the general population. Cigarettes were smoked by 64 percent of the bisexual women and 43 percent of the men, which is considerably higher than for the general population. Marijuana was smoked by 64 percent of both the men and women, amyl nitrate was used by 30 percent of them, intravenous drugs were used by 10 percent, and needle sharing was also reported by 10 percent.

It should be noted that in this sample, those requesting an HIV test are likely to have more health problems than the total bisexual population, so generalizations should be made with caution.

FUTURE RESEARCH NEEDS

Since the issues surrounding bisexuality in New Zealand are so under-researched, the need for further research is substantial. As a first step we need to know more about the size and nature of the bisexual population, its variety, and its makeup. New Zealand is a multi-cultural society so we need to research bisexuality among Maori and Pacific

Island groups as well as the majority European group. For the purposes of HIV epidemiological estimates and for the better targeting of prevention strategies, we need information on risk behaviors among bisexuals and changes in these. These need to be ongoing monitoring studies that examine both the meaning and the consistency of these changes, as well as their incidence. Of particular concern are the partners of bisexuals in New Zealand, about whom we know nothing. Among partners and bisexuals themselves we need to research exposure to unsafe sexual practices.

Another area of concern is the health and welfare of bisexuals. As a result of their marginalized status we would expect particular mental health problems such as low self-esteem and low self-assertiveness with their concomitant problems. These matters need to be researched so that appropriate remedial programs can be established if necessary.

The particular problems facing prostitutes, transvestites, and transsexuals are also in need of research. To date, the work that has been done with these groups has taken a very clinical view of the subjects and has sought to explain their "pathology." There has been no work on their general health needs, the legal problems they encounter, or the dangers they face.

Finally, there is a great need to undertake research *with* bisexuals rather than *on* them. It is crucial that research involve bisexuals themselves in all stages of design, execution, and interpretation of research to ensure the validity of findings. Furthermore, the needs that bisexuals themselves have for information should be acknowledged. Research topics that are initiated by them are the most likely to be successful, given their inside knowledge of the problems and experiences they face.

13

Understanding Bisexual Men's AIDS Risk Behavior: The AIDS Risk-Reduction Model

Susan M. Kegeles and Joseph A. Catania

Changing high-risk behaviors is the only means of preventing transmission of HIV. Yet it appears that large numbers of bisexual men continue to engage in activities that place themselves and their sex partners at risk for contracting and transmitting HIV. We have seen earlier in Part 1 how global cultural patterns affect bisexual behavior. This chapter concerns the intrapersonal factors that influence the likelihood that bisexual men will engage in high- or low-risk sexual activities. As public health prevention programs are developed, it is important to be aware of specific individual-level factors that should be targeted for intervention. For example, as seen below, simply informing people about how HIV is transmitted is unlikely to change many people's behavior. More factors influence behavior than does knowledge about transmission.

The primary emphasis in this chapter is on individual factors that make some bisexual men engage in unsafe sexual activities with men and women (e.g., beliefs, attitudes, perceptions of social norms, and communication abilities). This emphasis should not be construed to mean that the wide range of societal, cultural, and institutional factors associated with why some men engage in unsafe sexual activities with men and women is unimportant. These broader factors are critically important to be aware of when striving to understand and intervene in AIDS risk behavior. For example, poverty may result in a lack of access to information about safer sex and an inability to obtain condoms. Similarly, there may be laws forbidding the distribution of condoms and prohibiting men from engaging in sexual activities with men (which causes bisexual men to become a very "hidden" population indeed).

Our emphasis is placed on individual factors rather than societal-level factors for two reasons: (1) within any given society there is wide variation in people's response to the societal factors; therefore simply targeting the societal factors will still not yield change among all individuals in that society. (2) Prevention programs may be more successful in targeting the individual-level factors for change than the societal and cultural factors. For example, it may be easier to help people learn to communicate with sex partners than to alter the legal system or change poverty levels.

One particular societal-level factor that warrants special attention, however, is that of the role of social norms. There may be the potential to influence some social norms (e.g., the norm surrounding which sexual activities are considered to be safe or risky), whereas other norms may be extremely difficult to influence (the norm in a pronatalist-profamily society that a man's worth is measured by the number of children he has). Even for norms that cannot be changed, we may attempt to determine if the norm can be used to promote safer sexual activities (e.g., the norm that one should do God's work may be used to encourage disease prevention activities as a part of fulfilling one's obligation to God, or the social expectation that a man has an obligation to protect his family may be used to encourage him to protect his family by using condoms when he has sex with other men). Although social norms play an important role in organizing behavior into distinctive patterns from culture to culture, we contend that because there may be tremendous variation in the individuals' perceptions of social norms, it is imperative to understand the individual's own perceptions of the norms.

The AIDS Risk-Reduction Model (ARRM) (Catania, Kegeles, and Coates 1990) was developed to explain why people persist in engaging in activities that place them at risk for contracting HIV (e.g., failing to use condoms) versus making efforts to alter those activities. The ARRM is a useful heuristic model, indicating to AIDS researchers variables to be examined and to be targeted for change. The ARRM is currently being used at the Center for AIDS Prevention Studies at the University of California, San Francisco, to guide various research projects on young and older gay men, black gay and bisexual men, and heterosexual adults and adolescents. The ARRM is based upon previous research in the fields of psychology and public health and integrates elements from the Health Belief Model (Becker 1974; Janz and Becker 1984; Maiman and Becker 1974), the Theory of Reasoned Action (Ajzen and Fishbein 1980; Fishbein 1980; Fishbein and Ajzen 1975), "efficacy" theory (Bandura 1977, 1982), emotional influences (Janis 1967; Leventhal 1973; Leventhal, Watts, and Pagano 1967), and interpersonal processes (Burke and Weir 1982; Rogers 1983).

The ARRM identifies three stages that an individual may need to traverse to reduce or change sexual activities that place the individual at risk for HIV transmission: (1) the individual must recognize that his sexual activities place him at risk for acquiring or transmitting HIV and label his behavior as being risky; (2) he must make a decision to alter the high-risk behavior and commit to that decision; (3) he must overcome barriers to enacting the decision by eliminating communication barriers, seeking help when necessary to learn strategies to reduce risk behavior, and being able to obtain condoms (if he desires to continue engaging in intercourse).

These three stages of the ARRM are neither unidirectional nor nonreversible. For example, some men may encounter difficulty in changing their behavior with their female sex partners and come to relabel their activities as nonproblematic or reduce their commitment to change. In addition, the stages are not necessarily invariant. Some bisexual men, for example, may have male sex partners who are determined to change high-risk activities, and the bisexual men may acquiesce and therefore alter the risk behavior but may nevertheless not perceive their previous behavior as dangerous.

Each stage includes a number of constructs identified in prior research as important for engaging in "healthy" or low-risk behaviors. The ARRM postulates that it may be necessary for an individual to have some degree of distress or anxiety about AIDS to keep traversing the different stages of the model, although overly high levels of anxiety may hinder effective behavior change, and insufficient anxiety about AIDS may not motivate the individual to alter the high-risk activities. These constructs and the model are described below.

STAGE ONE: IDENTIFYING AND LABELING
ONE'S ACTIVITIES AS RISKY

The ARRM posits that the first stage in reducing or changing high-risk sexual activities entails an individual's ability to recognize that he is engaging in activities that place him at risk for contracting or transmitting HIV. Thus, before a man is likely to begin using condoms with his female partner(s) other than for contraception, he must recognize that both he and his partner are at risk for possible HIV infection. Similarly, to change his sexual activities with other men from intercourse to nonpenetrative activities to reduce the risk of infection, he must realize that unprotected intercourse is risky to himself as well as to his partner. Thus, to change his behavior, the man must recognize and label his activities as being risky. Several variables are hypothesized to contribute to labeling one's behavior as high-risk.

HIV Transmission Knowledge

Knowledge of how HIV is transmitted is a necessary but insufficient condition to reduce high-risk activities (Brandt 1988). Early in the AIDS epidemic, level of knowledge among gay men was found to be associated with engaging in risk-reduction activities (Emmons et al. 1987); however, this relationship is not necessarily found in longitudinal analyses of risk behavior (Joseph et al. 1987). Becker and Joseph (1988) have posited a threshold effect of knowledge, whereby information causes some people to alter their behavior, but other variables account for changes above and beyond the initial effects of knowledge. Although knowledge is high among self-identified gay men in industrialized countries, little is known about knowledge among bisexual men in either industrialized or non-industrialized countries. Since it may be that a high proportion of bisexual men engage primarily in insertive anal intercourse with their male partners, it is important that they understand that both insertive and receptive anal intercourse put them at risk for contacting and transmitting HIV.

Perceived Personal Susceptibility to AIDS

It is assumed that individuals must feel personally vulnerable to contracting AIDS before labeling their behaviors as high-risk. People may know objectively that anal intercourse is a major way of transmitting HIV, but for a variety of reasons they may doubt that they themselves are vulnerable to infection. For example, an individual may be aware that he has engaged in anal intercourse on numerous occasions but has not yet become infected. This may lead the individual to believe that his body is somehow able to "fight off" HIV. Alternatively, he may believe that he is particularly able to determine what kind of person might carry HIV. In either case, the individual does not feel personally vulnerable to HIV and therefore will not come to label his activities as being harmful.

Perceived Social Norms Regarding Perception of Risk

ARRM posits that what an individual thinks his reference group considers to be high-risk sexual practices influences whether he labels the behavior as risky. If a man believes, for example, that most people who are important to him think that insertive anal intercourse is not particularly risky, it is unlikely that he will define this activity as such.

Sexual Identity and Self-Concept

Both an individual's sexual self-concept and a recognition of sexual activities may influence the extent to which an individual labels his activities as being harmful. Thus, for a man to realize that he is placing himself at risk for contracting or transmitting HIV, he may either need to have a bisexual identity or at least comprehend that he indeed has "sex" with men. It is quite likely that some men who are behaviorally bisexual continue to identify themselves as being heterosexual. This may be particularly true in cultures in which sexual identities include only "inserters" and "receptives." In such cultures, it may be believed that men who insert are heterosexual and men who receive are homosexual. If they believe that only homosexual men are at risk for HIV, then men who are always the insertive partner may not be aware of the inherent risks of their own behavior. Similarly, a man might not construe his activities as having "sex with men." In some cultures, sex may only be defined as activities a man engages in with women; activities among men are considered to be something else. Thus, from the individual's perspective, since he is not having sex with men, he is not at risk. This points to the necessity of understanding sexual identity, sexual self-concept issues, and the meaning of sexual activities in a particular culture and society when attempting to encourage people to recognize their risk for HIV.

STAGE TWO: COMMITMENT TO
ENGAGING IN LOW-RISK ACTIVITIES

Given that an individual has labeled his behavior as harmful, two types of variables will influence the likelihood that the person will commit to engaging in low-risk behaviors: attitudes about high- and low-risk activities, and beliefs in his ability to enact low-risk activities.

Attitudes about the High- and Low-Risk Activites

Whether or not an individual decides to reduce his high-risk sexual practices is determined by his analysis of the costs and benefits (positive and negative consequences) of continuing that behavior and of changing the behavior. People hold widely varying attitudes about high- and low-risk activities, and undoubtedly these vary extensively between cultures. For example, an extremely important attitude among some people is that nonpenetrative sex and using condoms are less enjoyable than unprotected intercourse, a large negative consequence of changing from high- to low-risk activities. Interpersonal consequences of altering sexual activities may include concerns that the female partner will learn of the bisexual man's sexual activities with other men. Interpersonal consequences could also include instances where a male partner will reject the individual because he fears that the bisexual man is diseased because he desires low-risk sex. In a strongly pronatalist society, it may be considered "sinful" to use condoms during intercourse with women, since condoms prevent a female from a potential pregnancy. Thus, perceived enjoyment of the high- and low-risk activities, perceived efficacy of the advocated low-risk activity in achieving risk reduction, interpersonal costs associated with requesting a change in sexual activities, the perceived social norms surrounding the low- and high-risk activities, as well as other attitudes, are all likely to influence commitment to engage in low-risk behavior. In deciding whether or not to alter his sexual activities, the individual may "trade-off" the various costs and benefits of engaging in low- and high-risk behaviors. For example, if the threat that a man's female partner may discover that the man has sexual relations with other men looms larger in the man's mind than the risk of contracting HIV, then the bisexual man may not alter his high-risk activities. Another example would be that some people may believe that condoms afford little protection against HIV and, balanced against the other costs of using condoms, are simply "not worth it."

Self-efficacy

An individual may feel that the benefits of low-risk activities outweigh the costs associated with the low-risk activities but feel incapable of engaging in them. In accordance with self-efficacy theory (Bandura 1982), the ARRM posits that to adopt low-risk activities, individuals need to feel capable of engaging in activities that will prevent HIV infection. In some cultures there may be a fatalistic feeling about disease avoidance in general: "I will receive whatever fate God wishes to send me." In other cultures, individuals may feel capable of engaging in activities that avoid disease; but at the same time they feel or simply are unable to acquire condoms, or to resist their partner's desires for high-risk sex.

STAGE THREE: ENACTING THE COMMITMENT TO REDUCE HIGH-RISK ACTIVITIES

An individual may label his activities as being risky, may commit himself to changing the activities, and yet face insurmountable barriers to actually altering his behavior. The third stage of ARRM concerns barriers that may need to be overcome to enact the commitment to change high-risk activities. There are at least three variables that may influence the likelihood that the person will act on his or her commitment to change behaviors: sexual communication abilities, ability to obtain help in changing, and the individual's access to condoms.

Sexual Communication Abilities

To engage in low-risk behaviors, an individual may need to communicate his desires to his sexual partner(s). Communicating about sexual desires may be very difficult indeed. A man, for example, may be committed to having his male partner use condoms, but if he lacks the social skills necessary to communicate this to his partner he will be unable to act on his intention.

Help-Seeking

People may seek informal help and social support from friends and family or professional help from a health-care provider to reduce risk behavior. For example, help may be sought in learning how to communicate desires to one's sex partner, in discovering enjoyable alternatives to high-risk sexual behaviors, or in finding out where to obtain condoms.

Ability to Obtain Condoms

If one chooses to continue engaging in penetrative sexual activities, one needs to be able to obtain condoms. However, in some countries condoms are illegal, whereas in others they are extremely expensive and therefore beyond the financial means of many individuals. In other cultures, condoms may be accessible in theory but are stigmatized and require an individual to request them publicly (an extremely embarrassing proposition for many people).

SUMMARY AND CONCLUSION

With the three stages of the ARRM in mind (labeling, commitment, and overcoming barriers), it is important to realize that changing AIDS risk behavior may be a process that an individual goes through, rather than something that happens all at once. For example, it may take some time for an individual to recognize fully that he is at risk for HIV, and he may not have yet committed himself to change. Another individual may realize that his activities have placed him at risk for HIV and he may have made the commitment to change, but he may still be striving to surmount various barriers to enacting the change. Thus, program developers should not interpret a lack of behavioral change to be an indication that the prevention program has failed; instead they should understand that they may have started individuals on the change process.

From this analysis of factors involved in risk behavior, it is also clear that intervention programs need to be developed to address all three stages and the various factors within the stages. For example, if a program only intends to raise awareness of the risks of HIV, or has as its goal helping people to realize that condoms prevent the spread of HIV, it should not be surprising to find relatively little behavior change.

It is imperative that before (or concurrently with) developing prevention programs for different communities, cultures, and countries, research must be conducted to better understand the factors involved with AIDS risk behavior among bisexual men. There may be enormous differences in the precise nature of the three stages between different countries and cultures. For example, a program developed with respect to specific attitudes and social norms about sexual activities in one culture may fail in another culture where people hold different attitudes and other social norms prevail. Bisexual men throughout the world continue to contract HIV and transmit it to their partners. These men may face far more stigmatization and receive far less support from society in general, and from their own social circles, than homosexual men do. Prevention programs must be developed to assist these men in changing their high-risk sexual activities. However, as a preliminary stage to help bisexual men, we must first embark upon a basic research agenda to better understand the phenomenon of male bisexuality, and the factors relating to risk behavior and risk reduction in various countries and cultures.

Part 2

A Thematic Survey of Bisexuality and HIV/AIDS

14

Bisexuality and
HIV/AIDS Prevention Activities

Hans Moerkerk and Hans Elbers

In most European and North American countries confronted with the AIDS epidemic, attention was first directed to groups with an increased risk for HIV infection such as "men who have sex with men" and "intravenous drug users." In practice it meant that most attention was paid to those men who identified themselves as homosexual, since it was the gay organizations and gay men working in health services who took the initiative in starting HIV-prevention activities (Moerkerk 1988).

Those men who do not want to be addressed as explicitly homosexual or do not consider themselves as such usually are ignored in specific actions for "men who have sex with men" because they are difficult to identify and to reach. The same can be said for young boys in the process of "coming out."

Often it was considered sufficient to include items on homosexuality or bisexuality in relation to HIV infection in campaigns directed to the general public, assuming that married men with occasional homosexual contacts would understand the message.

THE EXAMPLE FROM THE NETHERLANDS

The Netherlands was the first European country with an integrated approach to AIDS, establishing its strategy in 1983 (WHO 1989). The first practical step was a campaign by the Health Ministry, public health organizations, blood banks, and homosexual organizations to ensure that donated blood be free of HIV. At the same time an extensive campaign was organized to inform the target group of "men with homosexual contacts" about AIDS to promote long-term changes in sexual behavior.

This first campaign resulted in the establishment of a national Coordination Team on AIDS (task force) with its own executive office. In this team representatives of the health authorities, of groups at risk and their health-care workers, blood banks, and the health education office, as well as observers of the Health Ministry, met monthly to ensure a national policy on AIDS prevention, care, and legal matters, also including nondiscrimination as an important objective.

The Coordination Team started as a private initiative with government involvement and has, in 1987, been reorganized as the official National Commission on AIDS Control. This committee also represents people with AIDS and other patient groups.

Activities in the Netherlands are divided among three target groups: the general public, occupational groups involved with the AIDS problem, and current (or potential) groups at risk. The last was defined as "men with homosexual contacts," "intravenous drug users," "the sexual partners of both groups," and "heterosexual people with (potential) riskful behavior."

In the Planning Model (see fig. 1), one can see how, since 1983, all activities directed to *exposed groups*, other *target groups*, and the *general public* have been carefully incorporated in a step-by-step approach in which *health information* and *health education* have been separated as different levels of a health communication strategy. Of course, those two levels are strongly connected with each other, as can been seen in the Planning Model; in a long-term strategy, however, it is necessary to make a distinction between *information with the bare facts* and *education* aimed at behavioral adaptation. To educate one first needs the facts. Within many AIDS prevention activities those two elements have been mixed up too much (Moerkerk 1987).

With regard to the largest group at risk, i.e., "men with homosexual contacts," the prevention activities could be aimed at three levels. These are called the three steps of the persuasion process: *behavioral change*,

FIGURE 1

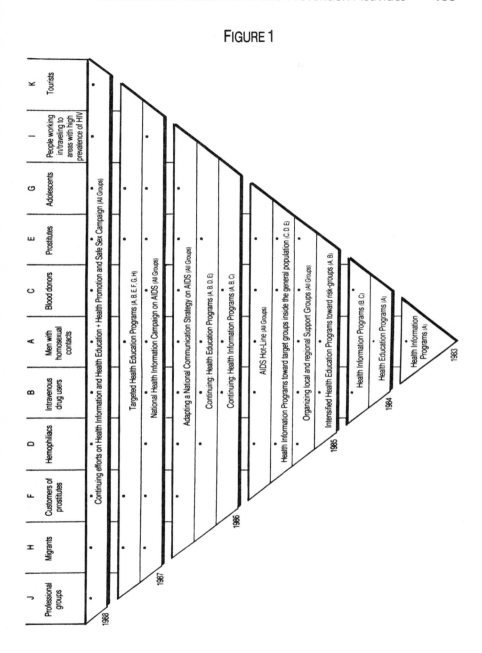

AIDS: Prevention, Information, and Education for Health;
a model of a comprehensive strategy used in the Netherlands.

change in lifestyle, and *subcultural change* (AIDS Coordination Team of the Netherlands 1987).

It is a step-by-step approach working toward achieving long-term effects by aiming at "modification of existing behavior" (using a condom during anal intercourse = behavioral change), "establishing safer sex as *the norm* in the gay subculture" (change in lifestyle), and "creating facilities and opportunities in which safer sex is not only the norm, but can also be practiced" (subcultural change). In practice this meant a fundamental reorientation toward the subcultural activities on the recreational side, such as contractual agreements between health authorities and owners of bars, bathhouses, bookstores, and (sex) cinemas to ensure that they would make their locations accessible for extended AIDS prevention activities. In the Netherlands, the authorities rejected as ineffective the use of repressive measures such as closing bathhouses and bars with so-called dark rooms. But with this approach it could have been possible to "label" a bathhouse as unsafe because its proprietors did not want to cooperate in educational activities.

This approach was not only advantageous for its step-by-step "dynamic planning," but also for its step-by-step evaluation.

AIDS AND SOCIETY

Preventive measures to control the epidemic are of essential importance as long as a definite medical solution has not been found. This means that in the future major efforts and attention have to be focused on a health communication strategy in which the general population can obtain concrete information and in which worked-out actions can be directed to target groups. Systematic and continuous health education plays a major role.

Health-related human behavior has been discussed as long as the world has existed; although attempts have been made to eliminate "undesired" behavior by repressive means and by declaring it "illegal," history shows that human beings will not change their behavior simply because it is desirable according to reason.

Changing human behavior involves a process in which positive messages must play an important role; this can be facilitated by *health education* and through the dissemination of *health information*.

Both health information and health education aiming at AIDS containment should be integrated within a general health-communication strategy that must be supported by a comprehensive health-legislation policy. The various parts of this strategy, as has been already explained, aim at *long-, medium-,* and *short-term* goals. Health education is conceived as a constructive and active effort implying multiple interactions, whereas health information may be mainly understood as an awareness-building process in short term.

We distinquish special target groups for those interventions:

1. men with multiple homosexual contacts (including bisexual men);

2. intravenous drug users who share contaminated needles, syringes, and other equipment;

3. sexual partners of members of these groups or of people from areas where AIDS is found in relatively high proportions among the population at large (Central Africa and the Caribbean).

HIV appears to be spreading rapidly within the first two groups, especially in the large cities of Western Europe, and in the general population in Central African and Southeast Asian countries. There are no indications in the Western world that HIV is widespread outside the target groups mentioned above nor are there indications that this will happen on a large scale in the very near future; even the possible links in infection between bisexuals and the heterosexual population will not contribute to a large-scale spread of HIV in the developed countries (WHO Director-General 1990). (Of course, this is no reason to abstain from prevention activities toward this group.)

HIV transmission occurs through blood-blood and sperm-blood contact; as to the latter, anal intercourse seems to be a highly effective mode of transmission when it takes place without protection by a condom.

The relative risks of other sexual techniques are largely unknown, although considering the results of epidemiological studies (Piot et al. 1989) they seem significantly smaller than for anal sexual contact, with the exception of genito-genital (peno-vaginal) contact between men and women.

Transmission by ordinary social contact, including kissing, is considered to be very unlikely. In working situations where contact with infected persons (or with infected materials) is possible, transmission can be effectively counteracted by relatively simple hygienic measures.

While efforts in AIDS epidemiology, research, and treatment continue to receive the bulk of allocated funds and political attention for the control of the disease, the less costly and standard methods of community health information and education should receive at least equal consideration.

It is the prevention of HIV-infection that will ultimately save lives and resources, and that can prevent anxiety in our society. It is the educational process that can provide the powerful tool needed to achieve meaningful and lasting changes in relevant behavior.

Health education is a process that bridges the gap between health information and health practices. An education process must recognize certain principles: behavioral changes occur voluntarily, the individual is ultimately responsible for her/his own behavior, and the individual must be treated with dignity and respect for personal choices. The result of a well-defined and clearly organized educational process is to facilitate individuals and groups concerned to make a clear decision on their own that will result in a continuation of (safe) behavior. Therefore, an educational process must offer a positive approach: to teach people what can be done instead of confronting them with what cannot be done.

A step-by-step approach toward both the general public and specific target groups is preferable because it provides opportunities for effective planning and fine-tuning its concerns to the needs of the society.

An aggressive approach that aims at short-term goals does not guarantee success. The message that has to be brought to the population, or segments of it, must lay a foundation for educational action. The dilemma in AIDS prevention is on the one hand the necessity to stop the spread of infection as soon as possible, and on the other hand the fact that effective results can only be achieved through well-planned and comprehensive action over the long run. A health communication strategy needs careful planning as well as a nonmoralistic approach.

Public health. This can be described as a system that emphasizes a number of measures that try to prevent the spread of diseases among the population or groups in the general population. In a Public Health Model two typical aspects are predominant:

(a) the attention that is given to the extent of the spread of diseases, and

(b) the financial consequences in terms of costs *now* and *later*. It concerns diseases that threaten larger groups of people or special groups at risk.

Public authorities. These must deal with the fight against infectious diseases that are threatening large groups of the population. They need to obtain knowledge about the extent, the areas, the ways of transmission, and the relationship with the social-cultural environment in which the transmission takes place or shall take place.

Epidemiology. This includes the study of social behavior and attitudes that can play an important role in the spread of the disease.

Prevention. This is the application of the acquired knowledge to create a situation in which the spread of the disease diminishes or stops. The process of prevention can generally be seen as a number of phases that can be adapted to the disease or disorder in question. Caplan (1964) describes prevention as the body of professional knowledge, both theoretical and practical, that may be utilized to plan and carry out programs for *reducing*

(a) the incidence (= the number in terms of time of newly occurring cases) of a particular disease (= Primary Prevention);

(b) the duration of a significant number of those diseases or disorders that do occur (= Secondary Prevention); and

(c) the impairment that may result from those disorders (= Tertiary Prevention).

This division into phases makes evaluation and measuring of effects possible.

Inside the framework of a Health Communication Strategy, as is described in this chapter, it is possible to focus on groups that are "hidden" under the umbrella of what is called "the general public" as well as on specific actions toward a target audience.

In the context of AIDS, this is particularly relevant for men who have both heterosexual and homosexual contacts. In both national campaigns and specific actions directed to gay men, gay prostitutes, prisoners, travelers, blood donors, and migrant workers, aspects of HIV transmission through bisexuality could be mentioned.

Table 1 shows *where* and *how* we tried to contact bisexual men and which target groups were used for that object.

TABLE 1
Access to HIV Prevention for Bisexual Men

Target group	Where	How
Prostitutes (male)	Gay scene, clubs, Street corner work	Condom promotion; supply of condoms; explicit safe-sex video and safe-sex stories in male pornography
Visitors of (male) prostitutes	Clubs, special information on the spot	Condom promotion and supply; safe-sex messages in porno films; safe-sex stories in porno magazines; special activities at meeting places
Prison inmates	Prisons, police stations	Leaflets and video promotion of condom use; supply of condoms; educating prison guards
Seamen, travelers, military, etc.	On-board ships, army bases, vaccination institutes	Promotion of condoms and supply of condoms; special leaflets and posters
IV drug users	Treatment facilities	Counseling and information, especially about secondary transmission*
Blood doners	Bloodbanks, general practitioners, hospitals	Information about sexual transmission (bisexual contacts, IV drug use)
Adolescents/street kids	Discos, coffeeshops, meeting places	Special videos; comic strips
Migrant workers	Working place, mosques, coffeeshops, travel agencies	Leaflets in 12 languages; special TV program; vacation information

*Secondary transmission is the transmission by IV drug users through sexual contacts.

To make sure that bisexual elements could be reached through the various mentioned activities, a lot of extra conditions had to be created such as the availability of special condoms for anal intercourse and detailed agreements with owners of (sex) clubs, editors of pornographic magazines, etc.

It also proved to be complicated to convince the advertising agency that runs the national information campaigns to include bisexuality in the items presented. This was of special importance during the campaign about AIDS in the workplace in 1988.

Although we could measure a certain kind of success with some specific elements of attention for bisexuals (questionnaires in pornographic magazines), it proved to be very difficult to evaluate the results of all those actions because they were included in actions aimed at broader groups. Since we decided not to make specific activities for bisexual men, it was obvious that specific results concerning that group could not be noted, unless general information made people clear about (bi-) sexual transmission of HIV.

Bisexual men, and especially those who keep secret about their homosexual activities, are difficult to reach; but with small-scale and creative activities, it is possible that this group also can become familiar with safer sex practices. Although these interventions cannot be measured on the level of assessment, secondary information such as knowledge about serological status* of blood donors, etc., indicates the relative success of these interventions. Being explicit is an important condition for all these educational interventions, as is cooperation with various segments in society.

---

*I.e., whether their blood shows the existence of antibodies to the AIDS virus (Ed.)

15

Bisexuality and Injecting-Drug Users

Michael W. Ross

Bisexual injecting-drug users are positioned astride a number of the important bridges for HIV transmission from one group to another. First, they are a potential conduit of HIV transmission from homosexual men into the drug-using population; second, they are a potential conduit from injecting-drug users (IDUs) to heterosexual people (Marmor et al. 1990); third, independently of drug use they are a potential conduit between homosexual men and heterosexual men and women; and fourth, they are indirectly a conduit toward vertical transmission. For these reasons, the bisexual injecting-drug user may play a disproportionately significant part in transfer of HIV infection between and across groups of individuals whose behavior places them at risk of HIV infection.

The link is exacerbated by the fact that a significant number of male and female prostitutes also use drugs, and that while males may provide homosexual sex commercially, they will often have heterosexual partners. Conversely, a significant proportion of female prostitutes who provide sexual services to men may have homosexual contacts. Confounding the issue even further, there is evidence that prostitutes of both sexes disproportionately use drugs. The use of drugs may be related to prostitution either through prostitution being a means of obtaining money to support the drug use, or conversely through drugs being used to make the commercial provision of sexual services emotionally bearable.

Boles, Sweat, and Elifson (1989) found that in the United States 13 percent of male prostitutes engaged in recreational sex with both males and females, and that 62 percent of the bisexuals (compared with 37 percent of the heterosexuals and 43 percent of the homosexual hustlers) had used injected drugs, particularly intravenous cocaine and heroin. Similarly, Chu, Doll, and Buehler (1989) found from an assessment of CDC (Centers for Disease Control) data in the United States that bisexual men with AIDS were more than twice as likely to have injected drugs than homosexual men (and that this did not differ significantly by race or ethnicity).

There is some evidence to support the risks associated with sexual transmission of HIV in IDUs in the United States. Donoghoe et al. (1989) report that IDUs at a needle-exchange station did not use condoms for sexual activity up to 79 percent of the time, and Jones and Vlahov (1990) report similar figures. Further, Battjes, Pickens, and Amsel (1989) noted that equipment sharing by male homosexual or bisexual IDUs with heterosexual IDUs was a common and efficient means of introducing HIV to low-prevalence areas. Williams (1990), however, provides clear evidence of the HIV transmission prospects from bisexual IDUs. He found that IDUs under twenty-five years of age tend to have partners who are not themselves IDUs, and that this appeared to be related to prostitution. Of his sample of 131 in the United States, Williams found that 15 percent reported sexual contact with both sexes in the past six months. Of those young adults who had had sex in that period, 38 percent had exchanged sex for money. The majority of male prostitutes reported that their sexual identity was strictly heterosexual and that they had relationships with young women who were also frequently IDUs and prostitutes. He suggests that contact with non-IDU populations through young female prostitutes' sharing needles as well as through bisexual clients of male prostitutes is a simple and direct one. These data confirm the special place that bisexual individuals may have as a conduit, through multiple-risk behaviors and multiple contacts, in HIV transmission.

The only study that has looked at sexual behavior in IDUs was carried out by Ross et al. (n.d.). They report on a study of over 1,200 IDUs both in and out of treatment in Australia. Of their sample, sexual behavior (as measured by gender of sexual partners in the past five years) was for male respondents, 81 percent, heterosexual; 13 percent, bisexual; and 6 percent, homosexual. For the female respondents, 68 percent were heterosexual; 29 percent, bisexual; and 3 percent, homosexual. These data emphasize, particularly for females, the high prevalence of bisexual behavior in injecting-drug users. Emphasizing the potential for HIV transmission through bisexuals, while only 13 percent of the heterosexual women and 10 percent of the homosexual women had been paid for sex, 35 percent of the bisexual women had worked as prostitutes. The comparable figures for males being paid for sex were heterosexual, 4 percent; bisexual, 34 percent; and homosexual, 33 percent. Further, the data suggesting that unsafe sex is common among injecting-drug users were confirmed by these data: bisexual men had unsafe sex 69 percent of the time (compared with 27 percent for heterosexual and 26 percent for homosexual men). Bisexual women reported unsafe sex 71 percent of the time (compared with 10 percent for heterosexual and 28 percent for homosexual women).

These data not only confirm the suggestion of earlier studies that bisexuality among injecting-drug users is associated with the risk of transmission of HIV to populations with low HIV prevalence, but also suggest that bisexual men and women actually engage in more sexual-risk behaviors. The disproportionate risks associated with bisexual IDUs appear to be associated with, in the case of women, increased prevalence of prostitution, and, in the case of both men and women, increased prevalence of unsafe sex.

While the literature to date on the area of bisexuality in IDUs is sketchy, with the exception of the study by Ross et al., it is clear that first, bisexual IDUs are in a unique position at the intersection of a number of risk behaviors to transmit HIV to presently low-prevalence populations and to act as bridges between populations at potential risk of infection. Second, the data to date demonstrate that bisexual injecting-drug users constitute a significant proportion of IDUs (particularly of female IDUs). Third, and of greater concern, the data also demonstrate that it is the bisexual IDUs who are taking the greatest sexual risks in terms of their unsafe sexual practices. Taken together, these strands of evidence suggest that bisexual IDUs, out of all proportion to their numbers, have the major potential for HIV transmission through bisexual behavior. A major focus of future research and AIDS prevention strategies on bisexual IDUs may well be one of the most cost-effective, as well as one of the most timely, in prevention of the spread of HIV.

16

HIV/AIDS Risks for Bisexual Adolescents

Robert B. Hays and Susan M. Kegeles

In this chapter, we discuss the variety of forms that adolescent bisexuality can take, review factors that place bisexual adolescents at high risk for acquiring and transmitting HIV, and highlight critical issues that must be addressed for HIV prevention with this population. By "bisexual adolescents," we mean adolescents who engage in sexual activity with members of both sexes, regardless of the individuals' subjective sense of their sexual identity, self-labeling of their behavior, the frequency of their sexual activity, or previous sexual history. Although we ignore those facets for purposes of definition, as we will discuss, those factors are of critical importance in terms of HIV awareness and prevention approaches with this population.

PREVALENCE OF ADOLESCENT BISEXUALITY

There is reason to believe that a large number of adolescent males engage in bisexuality. Kinsey, Pomeroy, and Martin (1948) found that 60 percent of males in their United States sample reported some homosexual experience by age fifteen. In Sorenson's (1973) survey of teenage sexuality, 17 percent of the males reported at least one homosexual experience. Carrier (1988) has stated that among Mexican adolescents the percentage may be as high as 30 percent. In an interview study of gay-identified youth in the United States (Roesler and Deisher 1972), the median age of first homosexual experience was found to be fourteen, with 60 percent of the males also reporting having had at least one heterosexual experience to orgasm. Similarly, another study of gay-identified youth found that 50 percent of the males reported having had heterosexual sex, with an average of six female partners (Remafedi 1987b).

Unfortunately, very little empirical data exist on bisexual adolescents. Surveying adolescents who engage in bisexuality is hampered by their lack of visibility and the social stigma attached to homosexuality that motivates them to remain hidden; therefore, obtaining representative samples of bisexual adolescents is extremely difficult. Further, the scant literature that does exist on bisexual adolescents has significant limitations. First, most researchers combine gay and bisexual adolescents into a single data set and rarely analyze bisexuals separately; thus potentially important differences between gays and bisexuals are obscured. Second, research on gay and bisexual youth often consists of adults' retrospective accounts. This is problematic not only because of the distortions and biases inherent in retrospective data, but also due to historical changes—in particular, the advent of AIDS—that renders adults' experiences less relevant to today's youth. Third, data obtained from adolescents typically come from specialized groups (e.g., members of gay-identified groups, individuals seeking mental health services) that do not reflect the diversity of adolescents who engage in bisexuality. Finally, while it is clear that both the experience of adolescence and the societal response to bisexuality vary considerably in different cultures, very little cross-cultural data is available on bisexual adolescents.

HIV RISKS OF BISEXUAL ADOLESCENTS

Evidence from a variety of sources suggests that bisexual adolescents are at high risk for HIV infection. According to the United States Centers for Disease Control (1989a), adolescents account for 5 percent of the AIDS cases in the United States, and young adults ages twenty-five to twenty-nine, most of whom were infected during adolescence, account for another 16 percent. The prevalence of HIV among teens is unknown and may be much higher than these data indicate. In studies of gay and bisexual men in the United States, younger age consistently emerges as a significant predictor of engaging in high-risk sexual behaviors

(Ekstrand and Coates 1990). In an Australian survey comparing younger and older men, fewer young gay and bisexual males reported having made behavior changes as a result of AIDS (Millan and Ross 1987). In a cross-cultural survey conducted in Sweden, Finland, Ireland, and Australia, Ross (1988) found that gay and bisexual youth reported a greater preference for receptive anal intercourse (the highest-risk sexual activity for acquiring HIV) and were more likely to have contracted gonorrhea than were older men. Similarly, among the gay and bisexual adolescents surveyed by Remafedi (1987a), 45 percent reported a history of sexually transmitted diseases. Adolescents who are sexually active are also more likely to use drugs (Donovan and Jessor 1985; Zabin et al. 1986). Although the frequency of intravenous drug use among teens is unknown, large numbers have used cocaine, stimulants, and other opiates, all of which can be used intravenously (Johnson et al. 1985). Thus, adolescents may contract HIV through sharing IV drug needles and then transmit it to sexual partners through unprotected intercourse.

FORMS OF ADOLESCENT BISEXUALITY

It is important to recognize that a variety of psychological, situational, and cultural factors may lead to adolescent males engaging in bisexuality; thus bisexual adolescents are a very diverse group of individuals. During early adolescence, it is quite common for males to engage in sexual play, curious body exploration, and mutual masturbation with other males as a way of experimenting with sex in a nonthreatening way. For example, Parker (1988) describes the widely practiced game of *troca-troca* among Brazilian males in which boys take turns performing anal intercourse on each other. Such experiences are typically viewed as a "passing phase" that serves as a prelude to heterosexual sex, and males who engage in this sex play are unlikely to consider their behavior as "homosexual" or to label themselves as "bisexual."

Engaging in sex with other males can also serve as a sexual outlet for heterosexually identified adolescents who do not have access to female sex partners. In cultures with strong prohibitions against engaging in sex with unmarried females, adolescent males often turn to each other to relieve their sexual desires yet would not consider themselves bisexual. Likewise, homosexual experiences are common among adolescent males in all-male settings such as boarding schools, detention homes, summer camps, or where females are unavailable. Depending in part on the meaning and stigma attached to homosexual behavior within the culture, individuals will differ in their emotional responses to these experiences. Some males may feel considerable emotional conflict and worry over whether the experience means they are "homosexual"; others may attribute their behavior to situational factors and dismiss it. As Carrier (1988) discusses, in Mexican culture, being the "inserter" in anal intercourse is not considered "homosexual"; thus males have few qualms about engaging in sex with other males as long as they are the inserter and their self-image as masculine and heterosexual is not threatened.

Bisexuality is also very common among adolescent males whose primary sexual attraction is homosexual but who are still in the process of "coming out" as gay. As Troiden (1989) emphasizes, due to the stigmatization and negative stereotypes associated with homosexuality, the acquisition of a gay identity is a gradual, often conflicted process. It begins with the initial recognition of homosexual feelings, typically noted in the period between early childhood and puberty, but for many is not resolved until early adulthood. During the period of "identity confusion," many males prefer to define themselves as "bisexual" because adopting a homosexual identity is too threatening and dissonant with the heterosexual self-image of their socialization. In the sample of homosexual adolescents interviewed by Roesler and Deisher (1972), 56 percent of those who had not come out described themselves as bisexual, although some had never had heterosexual sex. Seeking out sex with females as an attempt to suppress or eradicate their homosexual feelings is also quite common among adolescents (Rigg 1982). As several writers have discussed (Feldman 1988; Herdt 1988), the advent of the AIDS epidemic and its association with homosexuality have compounded adolescents' anxieties over adopting a gay identity and may further delay their coming-out process.

Some adolescent males who may personally accept that they enjoy sex with other males may feel the need to engage in sex with females as a "cover" so others will not suspect them of being homosexual. This is likely to be very common in cultures in which homosexuality is highly stigmatized or in settings where there is great pressure for males to follow prescribed social scripts (e.g., college fraternities). These males may have girlfriends or wives with whom they are publicly identified but engage in sex with males clandestinely. Situational bisexuality may also occur among gay-identified adolescents who find themselves in settings where there are no other available gay men with whom to have sex and so they have sex with females.

Economic factors may also contribute to adolescent bisexuality. Adolescents who run away from home or come from impoverished backgrounds may turn to prostitution as a survival strategy. In Allen's (1980) study of male prostitutes, 28 percent described themselves as bisexual, 19 percent as predominantly heterosexual. As Coleman (1988) describes, prostitution among adolescent males can take many forms, e.g., street hustling, working within agencies or brothels as call boys, or being "kept" by an older man.

For some adolescents who are experimenting with alternative lifestyles and behaviors, bisexuality may be seen as trendy or rebellious and adopted as a means of self-discovery or a way to gain status or acceptance among one's peers. Among British youth, this is exemplified in the "glamrock" and "genderbending" males described by Plummer (1988), for whom androgyny and bisexuality are socially valued. Likewise, Kelly (1974) has described the emergence of bisexuality among college youth as an "alternative adaptation."

CONTRIBUTORS TO HIV RISK-TAKING AMONG BISEXUAL ADOLESCENTS

A variety of factors may contribute to bisexual adolescents engaging in high rates of sexual activities that place them at risk for HIV infection. First, since many of the adolescents who engage in bisexuality do not identify themselves as homosexual, they may not perceive themselves to be in a "risk group" for AIDS. Even gay-identified adolescents may hold the perception that "only older gay men get AIDS." For example, in focus groups we conducted with young gay and bisexual men, participants expressed a stereotypical view of those who were likely to have AIDS as "older gay men with mustaches who go to leather bars." Young males may therefore feel it is safe to have unprotected intercourse with other young males who do not fit this stereotype. The prolonged incubation period of HIV infection feeds this misperception since adolescents who become infected are not likely to show symptoms until they are in their twenties. Thus adolescents may rarely see a peer who has AIDS.

Bisexual adolescents may lack adequate information about AIDS and safer sex. Research shows that adolescents in general are poorly informed about AIDS and safer-sex practices. For example, in a survey of San Francisco high-school students, only 60 percent were aware that using a condom during sex could lower the risk of getting HIV (DiClemente, Zorn, and Temoshok 1986). In their survey of Australian gay and bisexual men, Millan and Ross (1987) found that, compared to older men, younger males did not feel they had enough information on AIDS, and fewer knew the location of the local AIDS organization. AIDS education programs in heterosexual-dominated schools rarely provide explicit guidelines for engaging in low-risk homosexual activities. Due to their age, bisexual adolescents generally do not have access to many of the settings (e.g., bars, bathhouses) that may serve as sources of AIDS information to older bisexual men. Due to "closetedness," many bisexuals may not participate in events that are too openly gay-identified (e.g., gay student groups) that can provide an information network.

Because they are likely to be relatively inexperienced in personal and sexual relationships, adolescents may lack necessary interpersonal skills for negotiating low-risk sexual interactions. They may be uncomfortable communicating with partners about sex and may lack assertive skills to refuse attempts by partners to engage in high-risk sex. As Paroski (1987) found, gay and bisexual youth typically learn about sexuality by having sex. This may entail high numbers of partners and being open to trying a wide variety of activities with those partners. Among the gay and bisexual youth Roesler and Deisher (1972) interviewed, the median number of sex partners was fifty. These early sexual experiences are often with anonymous partners with whom they may feel uncomfortable communicating about safer sex. For example, among the youth Remafedi (1987a,b) studied, 30 percent did not know their partners before engaging in sex. Further, bisexual adolescents may not be sexually experienced enough to know how to make low-risk sexual activities enjoyable.

Feelings of invulnerability and immortality that characterize adolescence may also lead to engaging in high amounts of sexual risk-taking. When one is young and healthy, issues of sickness and death may seem remote and irrelevant. The less developmentally advanced cognitive skills of adolescents make them prone to egocentric or illogical thinking, especially with regard to highly anxiety-provoking issues such as AIDS and homosexuality. They may not fully comprehend the probabilistic relationship between engaging in unsafe sex and disease transmission, and therefore may not recognize the potential negative consequences of their actions.

Emotional turbulence can also contribute to sexual risk-taking.

Bisexual adolescents in homophobic cultures typically face rejection and hostility from peers and family and a barrage of negative stereotypes about their lifestyle in the media (Martin and Hetrick 1988; Rigg 1982). The resulting low self-esteem and depression many bisexual adolescents feel may reduce both their sense of personal efficacy in negotiating safer-sex interactions, as well as their motivation for doing so. Among the adolescents interviewed by Remafedi (1987a,b), all but one reported contemplating suicide at some time in their lives; 34 percent had actually made an attempt. HIV risk-taking may be a form of suicide for adolescents in despair. The high rates of substance abuse found among gay and bisexual youth (Remafedi 1987a,b) is also cause for alarm, in view of research that shows that combining drugs and alcohol with sexual activity increases the likelihood of unsafe sex (Stall et al. 1986).

The social isolation experienced by many gay and bisexual adolescents (Martin and Hetrick 1988) may contribute to their having high numbers of sexual partners, since sexual contact is often the only contact adolescents can get with other gays and may temporarily satisfy needs for intimacy and companionship. Engaging in unsafe sex may seem worth the risk to them if, by doing so, they can gain the partner's affection. As one HIV-positive male wrote in our study of sexual risk-taking among young gay and bisexual men (Hays, Kegeles, and Coates, in press), "Gay youth are incredibly in need of love and attention and oftentimes would do anything (including unsafe sex) if they thought they were getting that love and attention. I have a lot of bitterness over the fact that as a gay teenager, all I wanted was to be loved and all I got was a dick up the butt and the HIV infection. I got over it but it happens all too often to gay youth."

Finally, closeted bisexuals may be reluctant to use condoms with female partners out of fear that doing so would reveal to their partner they had had homosexual experiences. For similar reasons, they may be afraid to be seen purchasing or carrying condoms.

AIDS PREVENTION STRATEGIES WITH BISEXUAL ADOLESCENTS

In designing prevention strategies for adolescent bisexuals, there are a number of important factors to consider. First, one must recognize the tremendous influence of peers during adolescence, accompanied by a general distrustfulness and rebelliousness toward authority figures. In Remafedi's (1987a,b) study of gay and bisexual youth, 93 percent reported friends as their most important source of help with problems and worries; only 38 percent would consult their parents. AIDS prevention strategies that tap into the power of peer influence thus hold greater promise of impacting an adolescent's behavior than approaches that are perceived as emanating from adult "establishment" figures. Peer educators are thus a promising strategy with adolescents. For example, Arnold and Barnes (1989) describe an innovative program in which intensive training on basic AIDS information and communication strategies is provided to teen peer educators who then engage in street outreach to homeless and runaway youth in Los Angeles. Post-test questionnaires documented an increase in AIDS knowledge and behavioral intentions. Troutman and Hall (1989) train peer educators in AIDS prevention and improvisational theater techniques; the teens then perform original role plays and skits on sex, drugs, and AIDS for adolescent audiences. Featuring peers also serves to break down the stereotype that AIDS is not relevant to adolescents.

Protecting one's health may not be the most personally immediate or compelling concern for bisexual adolescents who may be dealing simultaneously with issues of loneliness, alienation, family problems, or substance abuse. Successful interventions may therefore need to tie HIV-risk reduction to the satisfaction of other needs for the adolescent, such as peer acceptance, enjoyable social interactions, or enhanced self-esteem. Indeed, one may have to entice the adolescent into participating in risk-reduction programs by embedding AIDS prevention in activities that are desirable for non-health-related reasons. For example, as a way to reach minority adolescents, Troutman and Hall (1989) have used a city-wide "Rap-Off" contest on sex, drugs, and AIDS, in which all entrants were required to attend AIDS educational sessions. Along the same lines, Cargill (1989) follows AIDS educational workshops for teens with a social dance in which the disc jockey and volunteers serve as "undercover AIDS educators." Free tee shirts, caps, and refreshments are also provided.

Given the stigma of homosexuality among adolescents, participation in prevention programs must not be socially stigmatizing or personally threatening. The programs must allow the adolescent to maintain the level of secrecy or privacy that he desires with regard to his bisexuality and to preserve whatever self-label he attaches to his behavior. Describing HIV risk behaviors without labeling them "homosexual" or "bisexual" is clearly the wisest strategy with adolescents. Likewise, tailoring prevention efforts aimed at heterosexual and gay adolescents so that they also discreetly and nonjudgmentally address the issues of bisexuals will probably be more effective in reaching closeted and situational bisexuals than programs specifically addressed toward "bisexuals."

In view of the undeveloped interpersonal skills of most adolescents, skills-training components that provide adolescents opportunities to practice skills necessary for negotiating low-risk sexual interactions should be incorporated into prevention programs to the greatest extent possible. Kipke, Boyer, and Hein (1989) developed a three-session workship for adolescents that effectively increased communication, decision-making, and assertiveness skills. In addition, since many of the adolescents most in need of AIDS prevention services may be disenfranchised from existing social institutions (e.g., runaways and prostitutes), innovative outreach techniques must be created to address their needs. For example, Griggs et al. (1989) use a mobile outreach-bus program to provide HIV screening, counseling, education, and provision of free condoms to young male street-based prostitutes in Sydney, Australia. Finally, any program that addresses issues of bisexuality among youth must recognize the extreme political delicacy of its role in most communities. It may be extremely important to avoid the appearance of "promoting" bisexuality among youth in the eyes of parents, religious, and political leaders.

CONCLUDING REMARKS

Gibson (1988) has described AIDS as an "accident waiting to happen" to gay and bisexual adolescents. While it is clear that adolescents who engage in bisexuality are at high risk for HIV infection, the difficulties and challenges of implementing effective prevention programs with this diverse group of individuals are equally apparent. A major impediment is the lack of empirical data on adolescent bisexuality to guide our efforts. More descriptive research on the sexual behavior patterns of bisexual adolescents is needed. Comparative investigations of the attitudes and behaviors of individuals who engage in each of the various forms of bisexuality described here would be extremely valuable in identifying critical issues that must be addressed for each group, i.e., their relative levels of knowledge about AIDS, feelings of personal susceptibility, motivations that may promote or obstruct engaging in low-risk activities, and skills for negotiating safer sex. In addition, methodological research on the most effective ways of recruiting and collecting data from samples of bisexual adolescents is critical. Finally and most urgently, intervention studies to evaluate the effectiveness of innovative AIDS education and risk-reduction approaches with bisexual adolescents are needed.

17

Bisexuality and Female Partners

Jean Schaar Gochros

Perhaps one of the few good results of the AIDS crisis is that it has increased public awareness of bisexuality. The first realization that the HIV virus could find its way into the heterosexual population via sexual intercourse between heterosexual women and infected bisexual men created instant panic in the American public. Stories sprang up about women who awoke after a sexual liaison to find notes pinned to their pillows saying "Welcome to the world of AIDS." While perhaps not panicked, many of those who, like the author, were aware of the large numbers of married bisexual men fully expected to see similarly large numbers of women enter the ranks of the AIDS statistics.

So far, such dire predictions have not come to pass. While AIDS in women has been increasing at an alarming rate, infection appears related to drug use rather than bisexuality. The non-drug-using heterosexual American public has settled back and somewhat relaxed, albeit with cyclical waves of fear followed by waves of complacency depending upon what popular magazine article has caught the public eye at the moment. Yet scant professional attention has been given to either the relationship of bisexuality and female infection, or to the unique psychosocial problem facing women infected by bisexual husbands or lovers.

This chapter will discuss the knowledge we do have, the gaps in that knowledge, and the research needed regarding actual infection and risk potential for adolescent and adult women, and issues surrounding bisexuality that are facing already infected women. Discussion will be limited mainly to the United States.

INCIDENCE OF BISEXUALITY IN THE UNITED STATES

Definition of Bisexuality

Bisexuality will be defined here in terms of rating on the Kinsey scale (Kinsey, Pomeroy, and Martin 1948). Despite inadequacies, Kinsey's study remains the most comprehensive and reliable research we have on human sexual behavior, and his scale remains the standard for measuring sexual orientation. This in turn leads to problems in gathering data.

True, researchers today are more sophisticated. True, even clinicians in HIV-testing sites are learning to ask about specific behaviors rather than group identity. Most studies on homosexuality, bisexuality, and HIV "risk" behaviors, however, obtain relatively small samples of people who identify themselves as gay or bisexual. Many such people decline to participate in studies out of fear.

Many men consider themselves heterosexual despite homosexual behaviors, and hence are either deliberately or inadvertently excluded from study samples. Until a large-scale randomized study can take place that focuses purely on behaviors and that also corrects Kinsey's cultural bias (i.e., he essentially excluded nonwhites in his research), we have little way of accurately estimating the number of bisexuals or the risk their behaviors may pose for their female partners.

THE INCIDENCE OF BISEXUAL HUSBANDS

Until recently, society all but ignored Kinsey's (1948) findings that 10 percent of white American men between the ages of twenty-one and twenty-five, and 2 percent between the ages of twenty-six and forty-five had had some amount of homosexual experience during marriage. Over 3 percent had had as much as or more homosexual than heterosexual interest and/or experience.

Again, Kinsey's research virtually ignored nonwhites. It did include hundreds of homosexual men who had had sex with older married men not participating in the study. Kinsey himself estimated the number of married men with some degree of homosexuality to be far higher (approaching 15 to 20 percent) than he could document.

Unfortunately, his figures again present gaps in knowledge about specific behaviors, with lack of differentiation between "interest" and specific sexual behavior during specific time periods. For example, it is unknown whether some young married men who had experimented with homosexuality prior to marriage continued to have homosexual sex during marriage, or whether younger monogamous married men may have, in fact, experimented (with potential HIV infection) prior to marriage. Hence, while his statistics clearly demonstrate a huge number of men who had had homosexual sex prior to and during marriage, we do not know just how large that number is, what specific behaviors occurred, or how frequently during a given period.

More recent research suggests that the number is large indeed—approximately 3–4 million at least (Ross 1983; Gochros 1989). Various studies suggest that approximately 20 percent of self-identified homosexual/bisexual men marry at one point in their lives (Saghir and Robins 1973; Weinberg and Williams 1974; Bell and Weinberg 1978). A smaller study (n = 200) by Humphreys (1975) found that over 50 percent of a group of men having sex in a public bathroom were married. In the Weinberg and Williams (1974) study examining 2,437 homosexuals in the United States, Denmark, and the Netherlands, approximately 17 percent of the men were or had been married; of that group 49 percent of the wives knew of their husbands' homosexuality, 16 percent "may" have known, and 34 percent presumably did not know.

Reinisch (1989) has figures based on a number of studies suggesting that 30 percent of the white American male sample reported at least one homosexual experience leading to orgasm after adolescence; 39 percent of both female and male adults reported at least one experience of anal sex; 70 percent of self-identified homosexual men over the age of eighteen had had sex with 1 to 5 married men, and 15 to 26 percent of self-identified homosexual men had either married or cohabited with women.

While studies and definitions of "heterosexual," "homosexual," or "bisexual" vary, the studies generally tend to corroborate Kinsey's (1948) original finding that no matter what label they choose, American men do indeed engage in both heterosexual and homosexual sex during their lifetimes. It is only the nature of that sexual behavior and the actual extent to which it happens that remain an unknown quantity.

Comparison with International Statistics

Although this chapter does not purport to deal with populations outside the United States, Ross (1983) cites various studies from different countries and eras producing substantially similar findings of between 1.3 and 1.8 percent of married men with some degree of homosexuality, and 10 to 20 percent of self-identified homosexual men having married at some point in their life. Around two-thirds of the wives had not known of the homosexuality when married, and presumably at least one-third still did not know at the time of the study. A positive correlation appeared to exist between proscriptions against homosexuality within a society and marriage.

Anecdotally, this writer is impressed by supportive responses to her study on wives of gay/bisexual men (Gochros 1982) received from people in England, Ireland, Canada, Mexico, Japan, South Africa, West Germany, India, and Poland. Her study and the responses to it included mixed-orientation couples from a wide variety of ethnic and racial backgrounds and from every major ethnic religion (i.e., Protestant, Catholic, Jewish, Buddhist, Moslem, and Sikh).

In short, despite gaps in knowledge about societies outside the United States (particulary non-Western countries), it is clear that homosexuality within heterosexual marriage is far more common than recognized and seems to transcend national, ethnic, and religious values.

Incidence of Sexual Relationships with Women

In 1973, Saghir and Robins noted that 48 percent of the homosexual men studied had had sexual relationships with women. Ross (1983) cites both American and European studies giving similar figures. In 1989, Reinisch found that the totality of reviewed studies raises that estimate to 70 percent.

SEXUAL BEHAVIOR OF ADOLESCENT AND COLLEGE-AGE WOMEN

Reinisch (1989) further cited figures suggesting that not only do both heterosexual, bisexual, and homosexual adolescent and college-age males engage in anal sex with other males, but adolescent and college-age women also engage in anal sex far more (23 percent) than was estimated even by Kinsey. Despite the threat of AIDS, approximately 29 percent of college-age men and women studied engaged in high-risk, unprotected sex with men both because of increased mobility in today's society, and because of the tendency to take more risks while away from home.

Seventy percent of college-age men and women engaged in premarital penile-vaginal intercourse. While space does not permit a more thorough discussion of her findings, they reveal sexual behaviors that place adolescents and college-age women at risk for HIV infection. Finally, she reports that 74 percent of the self-identified lesbians studied had had sex with men.

While we know that women continue to engage in unprotected anal sex, we do not know the extent to which that activity occurs with bisexual men. We do know, however, that many of the homosexual and bisexual married men cited earlier married at early ages, and that many of the older, married, supposedly heterosexual men engaged in experimental sex with women during their adolescence and college years (Ross 1983). There is reason to believe that many of the first American men to die of AIDS had become infected during adolescence. This writer's study (Gochros 1982, 1989) also revealed husbands having furtive, presumably high-risk sex during the very period (1970–81) when the virus was active but as yet unknown.

HOW GREAT IS THE RISK FOR WOMEN? THE INCIDENCE OF AIDS IN FEMALE PARTNERS OF BISEXUAL MEN

How concerned should women be about the sexual behaviors (particularly homosexual encounters) of bisexual men? Unfortunately, research fails to provide adequate answers and those that it does provide bring both good news and bad.

The Good News

The Centers for Disease Control (CDC) statistics of mid-January 1988 listed adolescent and adult women as accounting for 7 percent of all AIDS cases. Of that 7 percent, approximately 29 percent had been infected through heterosexual sex. Of that 29 percent, about 18 percent (26 women at most) had reported sex with a bisexual man. This was in comparison with 32,799 homosexual/bisexual men and constituted less than 1 percent of the total adult/adolescent AIDS cases. While CDC figures can change weekly, relative proportions still appear to be holding constant. In February 1989, out of 3,375 adolescent/adult female cases of AIDS, 1,025 were infected with HIV through heterosexual sex, and of that number, 100 (10 percent) reported bisexual men as the source. In February 1990, out of 3,837 total female cases, 1,023 had been infected through heterosexual contact, and of that number, only 96 (8 percent) reported bisexual men as the source of infection. If anything, then, infection by bisexuals seems to have peaked and to be decreasing.

The risk of infection from a single sexual experience with a man of unknown sexual history appears small. Many women who contracted AIDS through heterosexual sex became infected only after repeated—and one remained negative after 200—acts of unprotected intercourse with their infected partner. Moreover, many of those women could not be considered innocent victims of dishonest men. They knew of their partner's infection, had been counseled, and yet had disregarded the advice and warnings of their physicians and other counselors (Padian 1988).

As far as is known, *proper* use of condoms seems effective as a barrier preventing sexually transmitted infection.

What Do These Statistics Mean?

Do these low figures mean that most bisexual men have taken care to protect their female partners? That most bisexual husbands do not have intercourse with their wives? Or that most couples divorced before AIDS became a problem?

At present there is no way to know. One fact, however, seems clear: unless there are specific causes for concern in a certain situation, women do not need to panic simply because a sexual partner is gay or bisexual. Even if he is HIV-positive or has AIDS, that fact alone does not automatically mean that his wife or other female partner will be infected. Anecdotal experience also is encouraging. This writer has counseled countless bisexual men in an HIV-testing site, on the HIV team of a large military hospital, and in her private counseling practice. By and large, the majority of men, both married and unmarried, infected and not infected, have seemed concerned and careful to protect their wives or other partners.

The Bad News

That was the good news. Unfortunately, that's not all there is to the story. The primary bad news is that CDC statistics cannot give us the rest of the story. There are two major problems with CDC figures. First, until 1989, the all-important category of "heterosexual transmission" did not distinguish between five possible risk factors. Also, within a category—particularly in the large high-risk "drug user" population —are men who are also bisexual or who have high-risk homosexual experiences while under the influence of drugs. In the end, we don't know the actual transmission route for women infected through "heterosexual sex with an infected partner."

Centers for Disease Control figures report only diagnosed AIDS cases. True, a few researchers like Padian (1988) have studied women known to be at risk (i.e., have partners who are known to be drug users or bisexual, who are seropositive but asymptomatic), and/or who are sexual partners of HIV-infected men). These are studies on small, readily available homogeneous groups such as hemophiliacs or participants in a drug program. Married men, however, are often unwilling to either participate in studies or to reveal their homosexual experiences. When tested, they are often not asked about, and may not mention, their marital status.

Many women do not know that their husbands or lovers are bisexual and have not undergone HIV testing. Why haven't they simply shown up with AIDS? The lag time between infection and illness is a partial, but not fully satisfying, answer. As Randy Shilts stated to this writer (1989), by now we should have had enough monogamously married or formerly married, middle-aged women with inexplicable AIDS to demonstrate a "bisexual spouse" factor. It would be comforting to assume that such women remain uninfected. Recent studies, however, show an increase over the past several years in deaths of women in this category from a variety of respiratory illnesses in AIDS-prevalent cities only (Kaspar 1989). One must suspect possible misdiagnosis or deliberate failures to report.

The lack of nationally coordinated research on "seropositives" has prevented consistent and reliable data on exactly how a virus was transmitted (particularly when there was more than one risk factor in an individual), which sexual techniques were practiced, how consistently condoms were used, or how often condom failures occurred.

Stigmatization has created a "lie factor" that both interferes with reliable statistics and prevents couples from adequately coping with either the risk or the actuality of infection. If some anecdotal experiences are encouraging, others are not. This writer has also seen both uninfected men and infected men who knowingly and uncaringly endangered their wives' health through unprotected sex (with some wives becoming both infected and pregnant), and many who, afraid to be honest about their bisexuality, are taking themselves and their wives or girlfriends down potentially disastrous roads. Even when their sexual behaviors are medically safe, many men's secrecy (and often such safety tactics as avoiding sex with their wives) lead to behaviors and stresses that are hazardous both to the health of the marriages and the mental health of their wives (Gochros 1989).

Men are not solely responsible here. Again there is good news and bad news about women's—particularly wives'—behaviors. The good news is of empirical evidence that women are apt to be far less vindictive, homophobic, or suicidal when faced with a husband's bisexuality than men expect. Indeed, despite a variety of reactions, many wives are supportive, empathic, and flexible (Gochros 1989; Wolf 1985).

This writer's research and clinical experience (1989) suggests that the major determinants of a wife's reactions are not the anticipated factors of education or cultural or religious values, but rather the way in which the husband has dealt with and continues to deal with his bisexuality: his honesty, commitment to and empathy and concern for her, and the availability of an adequate support system with knowledgeable professional help. Clinical data suggest that these findings hold true even when the issue is potential or actual HIV infection.

The bad news is both empirical and anecdotal data (Gochros 1989; Hays and Samuels 1989; Padian 1988) suggesting that despite strides in assertiveness, education, and autonomy; despite increased knowledge about sexuality and massive campaigns to educate about AIDS, women —no matter what their education, cultural and religious values, or socioeconomic status—continue to place responsibility for their health and well-being in men's hands, often to their own medical and emotional detriment.

Also, the emotional upheaval surrounding disclosure of bisexuality may yield its own risks. Gochros (1989) found that dysfunctional, risky sex with either the husband or other men was a relatively common coping strategy or "crisis behavior" used by the wife to reaffirm her sexual attractiveness, or by the couple to reaffirm their marital commitment in the aftermath of disclosure.

PSYCHOLOGICAL CONSEQUENCES OF HIV INFECTION

Until recently, what little attention has been paid to female partners of bisexual men has often been more harmful than helpful, with wives' reactions to a disclosure of bisexuality or HIV infection badly misread. Even without an issue like AIDS, even supportive wives are often overwhelmed with problems of loss, betrayal, cognitive confusion and dissonance, guilt, self-identity crises, stigma, and isolation. They face both imagined and real stigmatization not only by the heterosexual and homosexual communities, but by unknowledgeable professionals and even their own husbands (Gochros 1989; Hays and Samuels 1989).

No matter what the infection source, HIV-infected women also face isolation and inadequate emotional support. When the issues associated with one's own infection and/or that of one's husband are overlaid with the issues associated with being the wife (or partner) of a bisexual man, the psychosocial problems are compounded (Kaspar 1989). In fact, the issues surrounding bisexuality may take priority as a source of stress over the issue of impending death. Nevertheless, both research and anecdotal data suggest that women can cope with honest disclosure of bisexuality more easily than they can *lack* of disclosure (Gochros 1989; Hays and Samuels 1989). Failure to recognize this can result in unnecessary tragedy.

For example, this writer was recently asked to help a "burned out" extended family cope with a demanding and labile wife with AIDS. Although the patient was seeing her own therapist, the issue of the already dead husband's probable bisexuality had been cloaked in a conspiracy of silence. Only when the issue was brought to light and resolved and feelings aired were the patient and other family members able to cope adequately with her own impending death. Unfortunately, by that time, the patient's own death was imminent. In the meantime, all had gone through years of needless anguish, guilt, a sense of "craziness," and loss of self-esteem brought on by sudden, total, and seemingly inexplicable rejection by the husband (presumably his own way of coping with guilt and anticipated stigma).

History seems about to repeat itself, in modified forms, with two other couples. One wife is already infected from a possibly bisexual husband. The other wife has voiced her suspicions, but her definitely bisexual husband refuses to tell her the truth, convinced that "it would kill her." While this husband can be counted on for medical safety, both marriages are in trouble with no possibility of resolution unless the issues can be named.

SO WHERE ARE WE?
THE NEED FOR BETTER RESEARCH

In conclusion, we know and "don't know" many things. We know that the number of women known to be HIV-positive or to have AIDS because of a bisexual partner is amazingly low considering the estimated size of the married or once-married gay/bisexual population; the number of husbands apt to have been having furtive, high-risk sex during the years when the AIDS virus was active but unknown; and the number of unmarried bisexually active men.

What we don't know is how many infected wives, former wives, or other female partners of gay/bisexual men are about to become sick, or how many women have indeed died of unrecognized AIDS. We do not have a reliable estimate of the degree of risk from a "category." We do know that bisexual behaviors are too common even in supposedly exclusive heterosexuals and homosexuals of all religions and ethnic groups to allow them to remain unnoticed, lost in a perhaps anachronistic and false categorization system.

We do know that education about AIDS transmission is not enough to prevent both men and women from taking needless risks. Although space limitations have not permitted discussion here, we know that complex psycho/socio/cultural factors affect attitudes and behaviors both in preventing and coping with HIV infection. We don't know how to avoid extremes of ethnocentrism and wholesale simplistic generalizations in our attempts to be more culturally sensitive. We know that bisexual husbands have created needless anguish for their wives.

We don't always know how to help such couples, nor do we know how to get them to accept what help we can offer.

Finally, we know that it is time to stop focusing simply on body counts and T-cell distributions, to stop "not knowing" and take the steps needed to "learn."

IMPLICATIONS FOR RESEARCH

We urgently need, then, large-scale randomized research that truly tells us what people do sexually, why they do what they do, and what sexual secrets they keep from their spouses or other partners. We need similar research on asymptomatic seropositivity, and we need to find ways to help people feel safe in giving us the data we need. Perhaps we need a national and international sexual census. We need both quantitative and qualitative research on psychosocial factors in preventing and coping with AIDS, and on ways to provide better social/emotional help for individuals, couples, and families dealing with both AIDS and bisexuality. We need research that will help us explicate both cultural universalities and differences.

The financial, political, and cultural barriers to such research are obvious, particularly for countries that can hardly finance basic medical care, much less expensive research. A key element, however, is not actually the size of an individual research project, but its place as an integral part of a total system. In short, we need an international cooperative effort with long-term goals that can be met through coordinated, incremental steps. One might call this a "systems approach" to research. Our world is long past the point where we can be satisfied with simply a myriad of unconnected studies, so different in goals, designs, and methodologies that they are apt to confuse more than they illuminate.

HIV viruses in each locale and country seem to have been creative, coordinated, and cooperative enough to *start* a pandemic. We must be equally creative, coordinated, and cooperative in obtaining the knowledge about human behavior necessary effectively to *stop* it.

18

Review of the Literature on Bisexuality and HIV Transmission

Mary Boulton

INTRODUCTION

This chapter presents an overview of empirical studies of male bisexuality around the world. Bisexuality in this context will be defined in behavioral terms as sexual contact with both male and female partners either concurrently or sequentially over the course of a lifetime. Studies that give information on bisexuality come from a wide variety of sources. Two main approaches were used to identify them: a computer search on the medical and social science literature, using "bisexual" as a keyword, was carried out initially, followed by a systematic manual search of sixty social science journals and a number of monographs. The manual search included, on the one hand, both general and specialist anthropology journals and monographs to establish what had been written on sexual behavior in "developing" countries and, on the other hand, both general and specialist sociology, psychology, and sexology journals that deal largely with the "industrialized" world. For practical reasons, these searches were limited to books and journals published in English.

It will be clear from this review that empirical evidence about bisexual behavior is uneven and difficult to interpret. First, many of the studies in which relevant information is given were not written with bisexuality as a primary focus and, indeed, bisexuality was not used as a descriptive term. It was therefore difficult both to identify studies and to abstract information from them. Accounts of bisexual behavior were often frustratingly incomplete since the issues of interest in relation to HIV transmission were not usually addressed.

Second, studies relating to bisexuality come from a number of disciplines, each of which has a different set of concerns and provides an account on a different level of analysis. Epidemiological studies are concerned with rates of HIV infection in various populations and the rates of specific risk behaviors (and changes in risk behaviors) associated with infection and transmission. Sociological studies are concerned with patterns of sexual behavior in social groups and the social and material conditions that create them. Anthropological studies are concerned with cultural rules and meanings that govern sexual behavior and the institutions that develop in response to them. It is very rare, however, for studies to be available to examine bisexual behavior in any one society or geographical area on more than one level of analysis.

Third, bisexuality refers to a very heterogeneous category of people who are grouped together on the basis of one common behavioral characteristic. The differences *among* them in terms of the context, nature, and extent of their behavior may be considerable and of major significance to their role in HIV transmission. This is the case *within* societies as well as between societies. However, these differences tend to be obscured both by epidemiological studies, which group all bisexual men into one undifferentiated category, and social scientific studies, which tend to be very selective in the social groups they study, providing little sense of the *range* of patterns that exist in a society.

In summary, our knowledge of bisexual behavior in relation to HIV transmission is very limited. For some geographical areas, such as Latin America, considerable progress has been made in understanding bisexual behavior sociologically as well as epidemiologically. However, for many parts of the world there is little or no information on bisexual behavior. Overall, available evidence derives from somewhat disparate and isolated studies that have not arisen from any unified set of concerns or research agenda. It is therefore difficult to build up any authoritative picture of bisexual behavior and inferences about its role in HIV transmission must at present be tentative.

EPIDEMIOLOGICAL AND PUBLIC HEALTH LITERATURE

Since the beginning of the AIDS epidemic, a number of studies have been carried out on the sexual behavior of homosexual and bisexual men by researchers working in the field of epidemiology and public health. This is most notable in Pattern I countries (Europe, North America, Australia, and New Zealand) where rates of infection are high in these groups (table 1). However, in very few of the publications arising from this work has the behavior of bisexual men been presented separately from that of exclusively homosexual men. Even more rarely has the heterosexual behavior of homosexually active men been described. Thus, despite the relatively large number of studies that include bisexual men in their samples, we know relatively little about the sexual behavior of bisexual men in these countries.

The exceptions to this include work on Mexico, Brazil, and some other Latin American countries where it has become apparent that bisexual men play a unique and important role in the epidemiology of HIV/AIDS. Consequently, greater attention has been paid to bisexual men by researchers working in these countries.

For Pattern II countries (Sub-Saharan Africa and the Caribbean) and Pattern III countries (Eastern Europe, North Africa, the Middle East, Asia, and the Pacific), there are few quantitative studies of homosexual and bisexual behavior (Carael and Piot 1989). Such studies are difficult to carry out in any country and in Pattern III countries, where rates of HIV infection are low, they may be a particularly low priority. In African countries, homosexual and bisexual behavior are claimed to be rare and taboo (Pela and Platt 1989). While they are not unknown, epidemiological studies have notably not identified them as significant risk factors for HIV infection in these countries, and research therefore concentrates largely on heterosexual transmission groups.

Size of the Population

A summary of studies reporting rates of bisexuality in various samples is given in table 1. Wherever possible, these figures are for sexual behavior, though some studies report their results according to measures of "sexual preference" or "self-descriptions" (which probably refers to sexual identity). It is important to emphasize that these measures are of very different phenomena and cannot be equated. Bisexual behavior refers to sexual activity over a defined period of time; bisexual identity refers to the way an individual sees himself and the group with which he identifies; bisexual preference refers to feelings of attraction or readiness to act in a certain way. Studies that report measures of both sexual behavior and sexual identity consistently show little relationship between the two, with bisexual behavior considerably more common than bisexual identity (Fitzpatrick et al. 1989; Davies et al. 1990; Lever et al. 1989).

TABLE 1
Rates of Bisexual Behavior in Various Populations

Pattern I countries:

Study and sample	Criteria for bisexuality	%
I. General population samples		
1. Sundet et al. (1988) (Norway: random sample of about 6,300 men and women)	Men who have had partners of both sexes up to present	2.9
2. Winkelstein et al. (1986) (USA: probability sample of 1,035 men in San Francisco Men's Health Study)	Self-classified as bisexual and one or more female partners in last 2 years	10.4
3. Lever et al. (1989) (USA: 62,352 men 18 years or older answering *Playboy* Readers' Sex Survey)	Adult homosexual experiences "rarely," "sometimes," or "usually" (but not "always")	12
4. Ross (1988) (Australia: geographically stratified state —proportional sample of 2,601 individuals 16 and over)	Currently married men, male partner in last year	4.2
	Previously married men, male partner in last year	6.4
5. Forman and Chilvers (1989) (UK: 480 controls for white men with prostate cancer, 15–49 years old)	"Yes" to "Have you ever had homosexual intercourse?" plus number of female partners	1.5

TABLE 1 (contd.)

II. Clinic Attenders

6. Christophersen et al. (1988) (Denmark: 365 consecutive male VD clinic attenders in Copenhagen)	Sexual lifestyle	7
7. Kolby et al. (1986) (Denmark: 737 consecutive attenders at 4 AIDS screening clinics in Copenhagen)	Self-descriptions	28

III. Gay Community

8. Bell and Weinberg (1978) (USA: 685 men with same-sex preference)	Homosexual preference and heterosexual coitus in year prior to interview	
	White homosexual males	14
	Black homosexual males	22
9. McManus and McEvoy (1987) (UK: 1,292 gay men nationally, responding to questionnaire through gay pubs, clubs, and magazines)	Gay man reported current female partner	
	London	4.8
	outside London	4.6
10. DHSS* (1987) (UK: 3 waves of men interviewed in gay pubs and clubs (Wave 2 = 298 3 = 284 4 = 251)	Gay/bisexual man who has had sex with 1 or more female partners in the last year	Wave 2: 27 3: 32 4: 29
11. Fitzpatrick et al. (1989) (UK: 356 men who had sex with men in last 5 years)	Male partner in last 5 years and female partner	
	(i) in lifetime	58
	(ii) in last year	10
	(iii) in last month	4
12. Davies et al. (1990) (UK: 930 men who ever had sex with men)	Homosexual/bisexual men with female partner	
	(i) in lifetime	61
	(ii) in last year	12
	(iii) in last month	5

*Department of Health and Social Security

TABLE 1 (contd.)

13. Bennett et al. (1989a) (Australia: 176 men recruited by newspaper ads and from venues attracting "closeted" homosexually active men in Sydney)	Homosexual/bisexual men with female partner (i) in lifetime (ii) in last 6 months	 82 31

IV. Homosexually Active Men Attending Clinics/Taking HIV Test

14. Welch et al. (1986) (UK: 270 consecutive homosexual and bisexual men attending GU clinic)	Criteria not specified	30.4
15. Soskolne et al. (1986) (Canada: 603 homo/bisexual men attending 4 medical facilities over 4 weeks)	At least one female sexual partner in last year	16
16. McCormick et al. (1987) men with AIDS reported to PHLS to end August 1987)	Criteria not specified	16
17. Evans et al. (1989) (UK: 4 cohorts of homo/bisexual men attending STD clinic and wanting HIV test (Cohort 1 = 329 2 = 296 3 = 212 4 = 213 Total N = 1,050	Ever been heterosexual Female partner (i) in last 5 years (ii) in last year (iii) last 6 months (iv) in last month	Cohort 1: 67 2: 66 3: 59 4: 62 29 11 9 5
18. Collaborative Study Group (1989) (UK: Patients attending STD clinics in 7 [1986] then 14 [1987] districts nationally) South East Thames, 1986 = 428 1987 = 556 Other, 1986 = 654 1987 = 1291	"Sexual preference" bisexual	South East Thames 1986: 19 1987: 25 Other 1986: 19 1987: 23

TABLE 1 (contd.)

Latin America:

Study and sample	Criteria for bisexuality		%
19. García García et al. (1989) (Mexico: 1676 men attending HIV detection center in Mexico City)	Men declaring sexual relations with men, and female partner		
	(i)	ever	56
	(ii) in last 6 months		19

In Pattern I countries, "general population" surveys suggest that bisexual behavior is relatively uncommon: between 1.5 and 12 percent of men have sex with both men and women at any time in their lives. For this reason, it is difficult to investigate in general population surveys, and most studies that report rates of bisexual behavior are based on samples of homosexually active men. Community studies indicate that the majority of homosexually active men have had female partners at some point in their lives and about 10 percent in the previous year. Clinical studies give higher estimates, with 10 to 30 percent of homosexually active men classified as bisexual.

Bisexual behavior is considerably more common in Latin America. Carrier (1985) suggests that over 30 percent of single Mexican men aged fifteen to twenty-five have had sexual contact with male and female partners, and that 25 percent of gay men have had heterosexual intercourse in the previous year (1989). García García et al. (1989) report a rate (19 percent) of "current" bisexual behavior in homosexually active men in Mexico City that is twice that (9 percent) found in London (Evans et al. 1989).

Lever et al. (1989) report that in the United States bisexual men were less concentrated in cities than homosexual men. García García et al. (1989) report that bisexual men in Mexico had fewer years of education and belonged to lower socio-economic levels than homosexual men.

Prevalence of HIV

A summary of studies reporting rates of HIV infection in samples of bisexual men is given in table 2. In considering these figures it is important to bear in mind that only four are based on samples constructed on behavioral criteria. In two (Welch et al. 1986; Joshi et al. 1988) the criteria are not specified and, in the remaining two, the prevalence rates are for men who describe themselves (Kolby et al. 1986) or their orientation (Collaborative Study Group 1989) as bisexual.

TABLE 2
HIV-antibody Prevalence Rates
Pattern I Countries:

	Proportion HIV antibody positive	
Study, sample, and criteria for bisexuality	*Homosexuals*	*Bisexuals*
1. Welch et al. (1986) (England: 270 consecutive homosexual and bisexual men attending GU clinic; criteria for bisexuals not specified)	17.9%	5.1%
2. Evans et al. (1989) (England: 1050 consecutive homosexual and bisexual men attending GU clinic who wished to be tested; (a) female partner in last month, (b) female partner in last 6 months, (c) female partner in last year)	30%	(a) 5% (b) 10% (c) 12%

	South East Thames	
3. Collaborative Study Group (1989) (England: Patients attending STD clinics in 7 [1986], then 14 [1987] districts nationally; "sexual preference" bisexual)	1986 16.2%	6.0%
	1987 17.4%	9.5%
	Other	
	1986 3.4%	0.7%
	1987 6.8%	4.0%
4. Davies et al. (1990) (England and Wales: community sample of 930 men; female partner in last year)	9.9%	5.6%
5. Joshi et al. (1988) (Scotland: 1659 "risk" patients attending GU clinic in Glasgow; criteria for bisexuals not specified)	4%	1.5%
6. Kolby et al. (1986) (Denmark: 737 consecutive attenders at 4 AIDS screening clinics in Copenhagen; self-described bisexuals)	36%	14%

TABLE 2 (contd.)

Latin America:

Study, sample, and criteria for bisexuality	Proportion HIV antibody positive	
	Homosexuals	*Bisexuals*
7. Cortes et al. (1989) (Brazil: 128 homo-sexual and bisexual men recruited from bars and clubs; sex with both men and women in previous 3 years)	23%	28%
8. García García et al. (1989) (Mexico: 1676 homo/bisexual men attending HIV detection center in Mexico City; (a) male and female partners ever; (b) male and female partners in last 6 months)	35%	(a) 28% (b) 23%

In Pattern I countries, bisexual men have an HIV-seroprevalence rate above that of heterosexual men, but well below that of exclusively homosexual men.

In Latin America, seroprevalence rates among bisexual men are higher both in comparison with rates among homosexual men and in comparison with rates in Pattern I countries. Carrier (1989), Cortes et al. (1989), and Beach et al. (1989) suggest that given the high rates of seroprevalence among bisexual men, they may act as the "chief bridge" of infection between the homosexual and heterosexual groups.

Risk Factors for Infection Among Bisexual Men

Given the striking differences in seroprevalence rates between bisexual and homosexual men in Pattern I countries, it might be expected that patterns of sexual behavior would also be strikingly different. In fact, patterns of homosexual behavior among bisexual men are broadly similar to those of exclusively homosexual men, with only a minority of individuals continuing to engage in unprotected anal intercourse, more commonly with regular partners than casual partners (Bennett et al. 1989a,b; Connell et al. 1989; Ekstrand et al. 1989; Fitzpatrick et al. 1989). Within this general pattern, however, there is some variability between geographical areas and social groups. In a sample of black men in California, Peterson et al. (1989) found that bisexual men had higher numbers of sexual partners and a higher percentage of unsafe sex than exclusively homosexual men.

Among men using a telephone counseling service in Melbourne, Australia, Palmer (1989) found lower levels of knowledge of safe sex among bisexual men than was the case within the gay community as a whole.

The studies of sexual behavior among bisexual men in Latin America present a picture more consistent with the high rates of seropositivity found there. García García et al. (1989) report risk practices associated with HIV seropositivity to be similar to those described in homosexuals in Mexico. In relation to Brazil, Cortes et al. (1989) report relatively high numbers of partners for bisexual men: 4 in the last month for nonprostitutes and 19 for prostitutes. About half (49 percent) of bisexual men never use condoms.

Risk Factors for Transmission to Female Partners

Few studies describe sexual behavior with female partners. Those that do indicate that bisexual men have fewer female than male partners in a year, but that they are more likely to have unprotected penetrative sex with their female partners (Bennett et al. 1989a,b; Ekstrand et al. 1989; Fitzpatrick et al. 1989). The shift to safer sex that has been widely documented for male partners has not occurred to the same extent with female partners. Ekstrand et al. (1989) speculate that this could reflect the belief that unprotected sex with women is less risky than unprotected anal sex with men.

In their studies of community samples of bisexual men, both Bennett et al. (1989a,b) in Sydney, Australia, and Fitzpatrick et al. (1989) in England report a pattern of sexual activities with female partners similar to that found among heterosexuals: about 90 percent practiced vaginal intercourse (most without a condom); less than 20 percent, anal intercourse. These rates of anal intercourse are similar to those found among women attending an STD clinic in London (Evans et al. 1989). This contrasts with the findings of heterosexual transmission studies, which look at seropositive men and their female partners. These studies report higher rates of anal intercourse with female partners of bisexuals compared to other men (Padian et al. 1987; Roumelioutou-Karayannis et al. 1988; European Study Group 1989), and a significant association between anal intercourse and seroconversion in female partners.

Similar findings are reported in relation to Brazil (Sion et al. 1989): high rates of anal intercourse among HIV-positive bisexual men and their female partners (44 percent), and a higher rate of seroconversion among those female partners who practiced it.

A factor that may influence the use of condoms in penetrative sex with women is the women's knowledge of their partners' homosexual activities. Only one study reports on disclosure to female partners: Gallo-Silver et al. (1989) found that, prior to learning of their HIV status, only 11 percent of currently married bisexuals had told their wives of their bisexuality.

None of these studies provide any information on the female partners of bisexual men: for example, their age, marital status, or whether they themselves are bisexual or have other male partners.

Limitations of Epidemiology and Public Health Studies

Epidemiological studies have provided valuable quantitative information on aspects of sexual behavior and changes in sexual behavior that are relevant to HIV transmission and the course of the AIDS epidemic, particularly in Pattern I countries. However, these figures need to be interpreted with caution. Very few studies are based on random community samples, and most rely on clinic samples that may be biased toward the more sexually active, and perhaps the more urban and middle class, sectors of the population. Many use opportunistic samples gathered from the gay community, which may underrepresent those whose primary involvement is heterosexual, or from groups of HIV antibody-positive patients who may reflect one extreme of bisexual men. Criteria for classifying men as bisexual vary between the studies and in some cases are not specified. Most use behavioral criteria (e.g., sexual history) but the time frame chosen varies or is unspecified. Others rely on self-report of sexual orientation or sexual preference, though orientation and behavior are known to be poorly correlated. Samples defined by the different criteria are in no sense comparable.

The very striking differences in HIV-seroprevalence rates and in the patterns of sexual behavior reported in different countries point to the crucial role of social and cultural factors in shaping the epidemiology of the AIDS epidemic. However, epidemiological studies themselves provide little insight into what these factors are or how they operate. To understand these issues, we must look to the social science literature.

ANTHROPOLOGICAL AND SOCIOLOGICAL LITERATURE

In the social sciences there is a long tradition of interest in sexuality and sexual behavior. Most of this work was carried out well before the AIDS epidemic and does not specifically address either bisexuality or the detailed behavioral issues relevant to HIV transmission. However, social science accounts of sexual cultures in different societies are important in interpreting the epidemiological data on bisexuality and HIV transmission. They give meaning to the epidemiological category "bisexual" by describing the social and cultural rules that shape sexual behavior, pointing to the contexts in which bisexual behavior occurs and the individuals and practices involved. An understanding of these features, and the ways they vary between societies, is essential in making sense of the different rates of bisexual behavior and the different patterns of HIV infection described by epidemiological studies.

Four broad cultural groups can be identified, which differ in the way the relationships between sex (a biological characteristic), gender (a social characteristic), and sexuality (a behavioral characteristic) are ordered: Africa and the African diaspora (the Caribbean); the industrialized West (Europe, North America, Australia, and New Zealand); the Middle East; and Latin cultures of the Mediterranean and Latin America. However, there is again a marked unevenness in the countries for which research is available. No studies on sexual behavior were found in the literature search for many countries, and much of what has been written says nothing of relevance to bisexuality. Standing and Kisekka's (1989) excellent bibliography on sexual behavior in Sub-Saharan Africa, for example, reviews several hundred papers, but these are largely concerned with the sexual behavior of women and with issues of kinship and filiation, gender relations, fertility and family planning, rape and female prostitution. With regard to the West, sociological and social psychological studies of homosexuality abound, but empirical studies of bisexual behavior are rare. By contrast, bisexuality is a major theme in studies of Latin America and of Melanesia.

Africa and the African Diaspora

In the cultural traditions of Africa, where the desire for children is very high, gender is defined on the basis of sex and sexuality is linked to reproduction (Caplan 1987). Heterosexual activity is facilitated because it is associated with fertility, while homosexuality is seen as wicked and "taboo." Homosexual behavior is therefore likely to be rare and, where it occurs, to be limited to covert contacts (e.g., with prostitutes) or to contexts where heterosexual contact is difficult or impossible (e.g., "situational homosexuality"). Outside these contexts, sexual activity is likely to be heterosexual, which means that most homosexual activity will involve behavioral bisexuality.

It is not surprising, then, that epidemiological research in Africa rarely reports evidence of homosexual behavior, although this may reflect the invisibility of bisexuality, not the absence of homosexual activity. In an early study of forty men attending an STD clinic in Nairobi, one was "bisexual" but claimed to have had only one homosexual encounter, and the researchers comment that "homosexuality is uncommon in Kenya" (Kreiss et al. 1986). Where it is reported, homosexuality is generally of the "situational" type. Feldman (1986) gives anecdotal evidence of homosexual activity between white and African men and occasionally between African men in a Rwanda prison population. Hrdy (1987) reports an anecdote relating to a school situation and suggests that "pockets of homosexuality" may exist where older men have authority over younger men, as in schools, and in migrant labor camps where few women are present. Moodie, Ndatsche, and Sibaye (1988) provide an account of this in relation to "boy wives" of migrant mineworkers in South Africa. These young boys had left their villages to work in the mines; instead the youths provided domestic and sexual services in return for money. Homosexual activity took place exclusively between senior men with power in the mining structure and young boys recently arrived in the mines. Sexual activity was interfemoral. Young men who entered into mine marriages could double their earnings and so invest more money more quickly into bridewealth and household formation in their rural home.

The West

In the West, where the desire for children is much more limited, sexuality has become divorced from fertility and is much more open and free (Caplan 1987). Gender is not so much ascribed on the basis of biological sex as achieved through sexual behavior. The element of primary significance in sexual behavior in defining gender identity is the sex/gender of the sexual partner. Heterosexual behavior is the norm and homosexual behavior is stigmatized in part because of the discordance among sex, gender, and sexuality involved.

Nevertheless, homosexuality is tolerated and a distinct "gay" community, lifestyle, and identity has developed in most Western societies. This development, however, has served to strengthen the distinction between homosexuality and heterosexuality and militates against bisexuality. Among the general population, any same-sex activity continues to be stigmatized, while within the gay community, the homosexually active feel pressures to take a stand as exclusively gay (MacDonald 1981). The sanctions against bisexuality by both groups helps account for the epidemiological findings that bisexuality is rare in Western societies.

Such sanctions have also inhibited the development of social institutions around bisexuality. "Bisexual" is not an acknowledged social category or an available sexual identity (Paul 1984). Bisexual *behavior* occurs in a number of contexts but, because of the dichotomous notions of sexuality in the West, it is rarely labeled as bisexual and seldom leads to a bisexual identity. Blumstein and Schwartz (1977) note that for most of the men and women they interviewed, bisexual behavior did not give rise to a bisexual identity. Identity was more likely to reflect the individual's reference group or the subculture in which he was involved. Until recently, however, there has been no public reference group or organized community available to validate bisexual behavior or to support a bisexual identity. Most of those who engage in bisexual behavior remain as isolated individuals, having little contact with other bisexual men and being hidden within the homosexual community or the "general population" (London Bisexual Collective 1988).

Bisexual men are therefore very diverse and difficult to identify. Blumstein and Schwartz (1977) emphasized the heterogeneity of the men and women in their sample. Their sexual histories were "discontinuous," moving suddenly and unpredictably between homosexual and heterosexual behavior. Most came to a bisexual identity or pattern of behavior through sexual experimentation with friends, through "liberal hedonistic environments such as group sex," or through adherence to an ideology of humanistic libertarianism. In a study of bisexual men in the United Kingdom, Boulton et al. (1989) identified six distinct patterns in the men's sexual histories. Almost half the men did not think of themselves as bisexual and three-quarters felt that others did not think of them as bisexual. Epidemiological studies often fail to recognize this diversity within the category of "bisexual." Moreover, most epidemiological studies draw their samples largely from those active in the gay community, which represents only one sector of bisexual men.

In Western societies, bisexual behavior might be expected to occur in five main contexts.

Adolescence

Surveys of sexual behavior among adolescents in the United Kingdom (Abrams et al. 1990) and United States (O'Reilly and Aral 1985) show that the vast majority—65 to 90 percent—will have had sexual intercourse by the time they are twenty. It is often noted that in the course of "experimentation" teenage boys may have homosexual experience (without going on to a homosexual lifestyle) (Rigg 1982). Similarly, the sexual histories of adult gay men indicate the majority had some heterosexual experience as adolescents (Fitzpatrick et al. 1989). It might be expected, then, that bisexual behavior is more common among adolescents than other groups and that it shows its own particular features. For example, it may be tolerated more easily, being defined as "adolescent exploration" and have little significance for public labeling or for adult sexual identity (Warwick and Aggleton 1990). However, surveys which look at sexual activity among adolescents rarely ask about the sex of the partner and there are no descriptive studies of adolescent bisexual behavior.

Married Homosexual Men

Since the late 1970s a number of studies have been published on married homosexual men, especially in the United States. These studies tend to focus on issues having to do with marriage—for example, reasons for it, what makes it work or fail—rather than on sexual behavior. They give little indication of the nature of the men's homosexual contacts or the context in which they occurred, either prior to or during their marriage. Accounts of sexual activities with wives and other women are also vague.

More general studies of homosexuality give a fuller picture of married homosexual men. In such studies the proportion of men who are or have been married varies considerably, from 4 percent (Davies et al. 1990) in a sample drawn largely from the gay community, to 54 percent (Humphreys 1970) in a sample of men having casual sex in public toilets. In presenting the results of the 1970 survey of sexual behavior in the United States, Fay et al. (1989) note that half the men who had male partners in the preceding year were, or had been, married. The homosexual activities of these married men are generally thought to involve casual sex in public places. For example, it has been hypothesized that the clients of male (and female) prostitutes are married men. While empirical evidence for this is sparse, biographical accounts of male sex workers seem to support this suggestion (Bloor et al. 1990). Similarly,

Humphreys (1970) found that over half of the men using public conveniences for quick and impersonal homosexual encounters were married, and he stressed that there was no evidence that suggested their marriages were any more unstable than the norm. Presumably for many of these men, who may well make up the majority of homosexually active married men, such activity remains covert, stigmatized, and entirely separate from their everyday married life and their day-to-day identities. They may be particularly concerned to keep their sexual contacts with men hidden from their wives. For example, in a study of 21 women who were married to bisexual men, Hays and Samuels (1989) found that only three (14 percent) women had known of their husbands' sexual orientation before marriage. The other 18 women learned of their husbands' bisexuality a mean of 16 years after they were married.

Bisexuality

In the last twenty years, a more experimental sexual climate has allowed some people to "choose" a specifically bisexual lifestyle (London Bisexual Collective 1988; Gagnon 1989). Virtually no systematic research has been done on self-identified bisexual men, however, and their social characteristics, their lifestyle, and their patterns of sexual activity remain unclear. "Bisexual groups" have been established to provide support for bisexual men and women, to foster the development of a distinct bisexual identity, and to promote bisexuality as a lifestyle. Such groups exist in a number of cities in the United States and Britain (Barr 1985; Mishaan 1985; Rubenstein and Slater 1985; London Bisexual Collective 1988) but they, too, have received little research attention. They appear to provide counseling, social support, and political organization for bisexually identified men and women, rather than a bisexual "scene" in the sense that gay pubs and clubs do.

Prostitution

Male prostitutes have attracted less attention than female prostitutes in relation to HIV infection. Little is known of the prevalence of male prostitution, the types and sexual activities of its practitioners, or the source and magnitude of the demand for their services. It is also unclear what proportion of male prostitutes also have female partners. Some studies claim that most male prostitutes are predominantly homosexual (Allen 1980; Fisher, Weisberg, and Marotta 1982; MacNamara 1965) while others claim that they are predominantly heterosexual (Butts 1947; Caukins 1974; Caukins and Coombs 1976; Ginsburg 1967). Two recent studies found that half (Boyer 1989) to two-thirds (Elifson et al. 1989) identified as heterosexual or bisexual, but this is based on reported sexual orientation, not sexual behavior. Elifson et al. (1989) also report marked differences in HIV seroprevalence according to sexual identity: 15 percent among heterosexuals, 31 percent among bisexuals, and 40 percent among homosexuals. These rates are considerably higher than the 8.3 percent reported by Morgan Thomas et al. (1989) for a sample of male and female sex workers in Edinburgh.

The extent to which male prostitutes engage in high-risk sex with their clients varies considerably according to workplace and local circumstances (Bloor et al. 1990; Coutinho et al. 1988). Recent research shows that, at least since the advent of AIDS, most sex workers do not routinely engage in unsafe sex with clients, although a minority report willingness to do so if the client paid more (Robinson 1989; Morgan Thomas et al. 1989). While little has been written on their sexual activities with female partners, it seems likely that they would follow the common pattern among other workers in the sex industry in not insisting on safe sex in nonpaying relationships (Day 1988; Morgan Thomas et al. 1989).

Situational Homosexuality

In institutions where men have contact only with other men, such as prisons, or have very restricted access to women, such as military establishments or schools, it seems likely that the incidence of homosexual activity among otherwise heterosexual men will increase. In all such institutions it is very hard to study homosexual behavior since it is both illegal and the existence of any "problem" is likely to be officially denied.

Prisons have attracted more research interest than the other institutions, but most studies discuss sexual aggression or rape (Nacci and Kane 1983; Scacco 1975); homosexuality as an institutional problem (Irwin 1980); or the "threat" caused by AIDS (Coughlin 1988; Berg and Berg 1988). Only one study provides a systematic analysis of the sexual behavior and identities of male prison inmates. Wooden and Parker (1982) estimated that 11 percent of inmates self-identified as bisexual and 78 percent as heterosexual, though 55 percent of the "heterosexual" men had sex with other men while detained. Sexual activities included both oral and anal intercourse. Heterosexual identity was associated with being almost exclusively the insertive partner, bisexuality with being primarily insertive, and homosexuality with being primarily receptive. Since sexual activity does not officially occur, condoms are rarely available.

Research on military institutions is rare. The American army's routine screening program for HIV identified 58 seropositives, and Smith (1987) noted the striking frequency of self-reported bisexuality, recorded at 54 percent of the positive men. Unfortunately, the study says nothing about sexual partnerships and behavior among non-HIV-positive military men.

The Middle East

In the Middle East, fertility is valued but only with a partner of the right status. Female sexuality is limited by a strong emphasis on virginity and enforced by institutions such as purdah. Gender is generally assigned on the basis of biological sex, and both sex and gender are distinguished conceptually from sexuality. Sexuality is defined in terms of the relative age, wealth, or social status of the partners (Caplan 1987). Heterosexuality is expected among adults but restricted access to women means that homosexuality is not uncommon. Although it is forbidden in the Koran (Farah 1984; Bouhdiba 1975), there is a long tradition of acceptable male homosexuality in many Arab countries (Miner and Vos 1960). So long as they conform to appropriate rules for ranks and hierarchies, homosexual relationships are accepted and not stigmatized.

Exclusive homosexuality and homosexual identity are therefore viable possibilities, and a minority of men may live this way. However, homosexuality is more commonly seen as a life-cycle option, and a *majority* of men may engage in homosexual relationships at some stage in their lives. "Lifetime bisexuality" is therefore likely to be common and to have little effect in creating a distinctive bisexual identity. Thus, as in Latin America, bisexual behavior could play a significant role in the transmission of HIV throughout the general population.

Only one study was identified that describes bisexual behavior in a society with roots in the Middle East. This is a detailed description of homosexuality in the life-cycle of Swahilis (mixed-race Arab-Africans) in Mombasa (Shepherd 1987). Homosexual relationships are ordered by rank, almost always between senior, wealthier men and poorer, junior boys. The relationship is defined in terms of the patron and client, and the client (paid partner) generally takes the passive role in sexual activity. The preferred sexual activity is anal intercourse (Standing and Kisekka 1989).

Bisexual behavior occurs over the course of a lifetime but different practices may be associated with different stages in the life-cycle. From the age of about twelve (when they start to move into the all-male social contexts of clubs, sports activities, schools, and social occasions), young boys are commonly approached by older men for sexual favors in return for gifts and/or financial support. These relationships may be for a single act of casual sex for money or for a longer-term relationship. Some boys continue to engage in such relationships for long periods of time, others return to it periodically when they need the money, and others move on to more organized prostitution. However, at some point most boys move out of this homosexual stage into heterosexual adventures before marriage. Since unmarried girls are highly controlled, these adventures are generally with prostitutes or clandestinely with married women.

Most men eventually marry and when they are sufficiently affluent may return to homosexual activity. As the patron in relationships, they now take the dominant role with younger boys.

The Mediterranean and Latin America

Latin cultures are similar to those of the Middle East in valuing fertility and restricting access to women. In Latin cultures, however, gender may be ascribed on the basis of biological sex, but it must also be sustained through sexual behavior. In contrast to the West, the element of fundamental importance in defining gender identity is the role taken in sexual relationships. Men who take the active role in sexual intercourse are regarded as properly male and masculine, regardless of the sex/gender of the partner. "Active" homosexuality is viewed with some indulgence and, so long as it is in the context of sexual activity with women, is not seen as inconsistent with a heterosexual identity. For men who take the active role, bisexual behavior is "invisible" because it is an aspect of normal (heterosexual) behavior, rather than "hidden" by stigma as it is in the West. "Passive" homosexuality, however, is regarded as feminine and stigmatized because of the discrepancy between sex, gender, and sexuality entailed. Men who take the passive role are regarded as "homosexual" and pushed toward exclusive homosexuality. In Latin America in particular, the relative unimportance of the sex/gender of the partner for those who take the active role helps account for the findings of epidemiological studies that a significant proportion of the male population has sexual contact with both men and women.

These men might be better represented as a subgroup of the heterosexual population than of the homosexual population, as they are in the West.

Reference to this sexual culture has been made in relation to Spain, Portugal, and southern Italy (Brandes 1981) and Greece (e.g., Peristany 1965). Empirical evidence about actual sexual behavior in these Mediterranean countries, however, was not found, and the extent of bisexual behavior and the contexts in which it occurs are unclear.

By contrast, the sexual cultures of Latin America have been described in particularly rich detail (Carrier 1985, 1989; Parker 1985, 1987, 1989). The links with Mediterranean cultures are clear (Lancaster 1988), notably in the distinction made between active and passive sexual roles. However, Latin American sexual cultures have their own distinctive features including a more central role for sexuality in cultural identity, greater sexual permissiveness for men, and more extensive interest in "exotic" sexual practices (Parker 1987; Pinel 1989). In contrast to the Middle East, where different practices may be associated with different stages in the life-cycle, in Latin America bisexuality may be a feature of sexual behavior throughout life.

For many men in Latin America, sexual activity starts at an early age. In relation to Brazil, Parker (1989) suggests that same-sex desires and practices have an important place in the experience of most young men. Among boys, for example, same-sex play and exploration is virtually institutionalized through games in which boys take turns in attempting to penetrate each other anally. This play is not expected to disrupt male gender identity or heterosexual interest. Mexican adolescents are also pressured to "prove" themselves through sexual contact with multiple casual partners (Carrier 1985, 1989). Female prostitutes and "available" neighborhood girls may be preferred partners, but "feminine" men are also seen as acceptable sexual outlets. The latter are more accessible and less expensive and so may be relatively frequent partners.

Once men are married, the sexual permissiveness accorded to them means that they can more easily and openly maintain extramarital relationships (Parker 1987; Carrier 1989). This is facilitated by the separate networks of friends that are important during adolescence and remain essentially unchanged by marriage. Married men may start or continue relationships with women or with other men, including male prostitutes. Unprotected anal intercourse is the most favored sexual practice. In some countries men are expected to be consistently either the active or the passive partner, though in practice the majority may be both. Condoms are rarely used, being condemned by the Catholic Church and associated with venereal disease (Carrier 1989).

Prostitution is common in the developing world, and in Brazil transvestite prostitution is a notable phenomenon. Virtually all the clients of transvestite prostitutes identify as heterosexual and the majority take both the active and passive roles in anal intercourse (Pinel 1989).

Other Societies

Other studies concerned with the issue of the social construction of gender describe an institutionalized "third gender" role in a number of societies. The aim of these studies is generally to demonstrate the dissociation between biological sex and social gender and to consider the basis on which gender categories are constructed and how they are integrated into broader social, political, and economic institutions. The classic example of such a role is the *berdache*, which existed in virtually every culture of native peoples in the plains of North America (Thayer 1980; Whitehead 1981; Miller 1982; Callender and Kochems 1983, 1986). The essence of their role was a *mixing* of aspects of roles assigned to male and female genders. Their sexual behavior also mixed aspects of male and female gender categories: they took the passive (female) role in intercourse with men but many also had sex with women. Because the *berdache* was both male and female, his partners retained their ordinary sexual identity, since whatever their sex, they could be seen as conforming to the norm of "heterosexuality." Similar institutionalized "third gender" roles have been identified in other societies, for example Tahiti (Levy 1970) and India (Bradford 1983; Nanda 1986). Wikan (1977) describes a "transsexual" role in coastal Oman, which involves homosexual prostitution. Such institutionalized roles might provide important focal points for HIV transmission were the virus to be introduced into a society.

Similarly, institutionalized practices involving age cohorts might form important avenues for transmission through a society more generally. A major example concerns male initiation rites in Melanesia (Herdt 1982, 1984; Creed 1984; Kulick 1985; Gray 1986). Young boys are ritually "grown" into men by consuming quantities of semen (the essence of masculinity). For ten to fifteen years, they engage in homosexual activity, first as fellators, receiving semen from an older bachelor, then as fellated, giving their semen to incoming initiates. Semen and masculinity are seen not as private property but as social goods to be distributed and manipulated in the name of male solidarity, prestige, and social reproduction. The roles of the two parties are best described as donor and recipient. The pattern of homosexual activity continues until marriage, after which it may stop or continue until children are born, when it is expected to cease completely. The final outcome is exclusive heterosexuality. It appears that "the males are heterosexuals who engage in homosexual behavior only as part of a symbolic process of masculinization" (Gray 1986: 66). Homosexuality in this context is highly ritualized, involving all members of an age cohort, and thus does not lead to a "deviant" identity or pattern of sexual behavior.

Limitations of the Social Science Literature

Like the epidemiological evidence, the social science evidence relating to bisexual behavior is extremely limited. Studies are few in number and highly selective in the societies and social groups they consider. Some are limited to accounts of ritual roles that are of limited significance in terms of HIV transmission. Others are concerned with "traditional" societies and neglect the way industrialization may be modifying views and altering the variability in patterns of sexual behavior. They can give no overall sense of the extent or nature of bisexual behavior around the world.

Some studies describe patterns of behavior and the social conditions associated with them, but few give information at the detailed level of sexual activities and even fewer consider safer sex and the use of condoms in particular. Information at this level is essential to understand and predict the potential dynamics of the AIDS epidemic. Anthropological studies often present their accounts at the level of the values and beliefs that broadly guide behavior. Many are not concerned with sexual activity per se, but with more theoretical issues, such as the social construction of gender, ideologies of sexuality, or the way rituals create and reflect divisions, solidarity, and hierarchies in society. The concern with cultural forms means they provide little quantitative information on the patterns of actual *behavior* in societies, which are the result of the interaction between cultural rules, structural (social and material) constraints, and individual psychology. There may be marked discrepancies between ideological constructs and actual sexual behaviors in a population, however, and it is impossible to make statements about the pattern of behaviors in any given society (or group within society) on the basis of accounts of sexual cultures alone.

CONCLUDING REMARKS

Further progress in understanding the role of bisexual behavior in HIV transmission will only be possible with more research on sexual behavior that specifically takes account of bisexuality. Research is needed in a number of geographical areas, including the Middle East and Mediterranean where bisexual behavior may be common; and in Asia, India, and the far East where patterns of sexual behavior among men are largely unknown. Current research in Latin America, Europe, North America, and Australia needs to be continued and extended. In each of these areas, more detailed and systematic information is required about a number of features of bisexual behavior, including the characteristics (e.g., age, social class, and area of residence) of men who have sexual contact with men and women, their sexual identity, and the way they interpret their own behavior; the numbers of their male and female partners over the short, medium, and long term (frequency of partner change); the nature of their relationship with each partner and the extent of the partners' knowledge of the bisexual behavior; specific sexual activities with each (class of) partner, particularly vaginal and anal intercourse; the use of condoms and other prophylactic practices; and the way these patterns of behavior have changed and are continuing to change in response to HIV/AIDS.

What has emerged most clearly from this review, however, is that research that collects detailed data about sexual behavior must also be sensitive to the social and cultural meanings of that behavior. Bisexual behavior is the product of culturally constructed sexual practices that differ between (and within) societies and shift over time. The meaning and significance of "bisexual behavior" and the context in which it occurs vary enormously around the world. These differences have a major impact on both the prevalence of such behavior and the way it can be studied. Large-scale survey research, with standardized questionnaires geared to the "general population," could obscure rather than clarify our understanding of bisexual behavior and its role in HIV transmission. Further research, particularly of a comparative nature, must be sensitive to culturally constructed sexual practices while at the same time collecting detailed information at the behavioral level.

Conclusion

Rob A. P. Tielman

The scientific study of homo- and bisexuality during the last century is an enlightening illustration of the ethical bias of many scientists. In fact, moral judgments against homo- and bisexuality were introduced in medical and psychological secularized forms. Fortunately, more and more scientists became aware of this hidden moralistic bias. Recently, the World Health Organization (WHO) announced that it would delete both homosexuality and bisexuality from the International Classification of Diseases (ICD).

Are sexual preferences determined by genetic and/or environmental influences? There is not enough evidence for an exclusive nature versus nurture position. The real question is: What difference would it make if the biological and/or environmental origin of, and influence on, sexual orientation could be proven? Neither nature nor nurture is an excuse for behavior we ourselves are ultimately responsible for. Justifications for our behavior should not be based upon the fact or assumption of its biological or environmental character. Biological and social factors can help us to understand how some events happen, but science can never replace ethical judgment. In democratic societies, legislation has to be based upon human rights, including the right to individual self-determination.

INDIVIDUAL SELF-DETERMINATION

In many countries discussions of sexual orientation are related to the tension between freedom and equality. Freedom can be interpreted as

211

the right to demonstrate one's preference which might imply discrimination against others, whereas equality implies the right not to be discriminated against. This dilemma can only be solved by a principle higher than freedom or equality. This higher principle is individual self-determination.

Self-determination means the right to give meaning and shape to one's own life as long as others are not unduly harmed by this. An illustration of the application of individual self-determination is the way in which human rights-based legislation guarantees the right to privacy and physical integrity, including the right to informed consent. No medical treatment can be forcibly applied unless to withhold treatment would constitute a danger to public health. This means, for instance, that it is against human rights to force people to take an HIV antibody test as long as the virus cannot be transmitted to others except in high-risk situations. No distinction should be made between "guilty" and "innocent" victims as long as everybody is aware of, and responsible for, the risks taken.

Better than the concepts of freedom and equality, the principle of individual self-determination is able to settle tensions between individuals and between minorities. Indeed, it is easy to understand why within pluralist societies the principle of self-determination developed as the leading philosophy behind their legislation. Countries having a long tradition of coping with religious, ethnic, sexual, and other minorities tend to be aware of the existence of diversity as well as more sensitive to upholding minority rights for everyone. Awareness of the need for minority protection is a guarantee for a real pluralistic democracy.

Based upon the principle of individual self-determination, democracy should protect human rights. By respecting individual and minority rights, including the rights of gays and bisexuals, democracy is strengthened, not weakened as many people assume. Majority vote is a necessary but not sufficient condition for democracy. The real test of a democracy is its fair and equal treatment of adults whose sexual behavior is deviant from that of the majority of society but who do not damage societal interests. For example, there are openly gay and bisexual women and men working in government, education, the police force, and the army. Research in countries like the Netherlands shows that a policy of nondiscrimination toward gays and bisexuals has not damaged society at all.

Tolerant attitudes toward homo- and bisexuality may or may not be a good indicator of tolerance in general. The Greek, Roman, and

Renaissance cultures were relatively tolerant toward homo- and bisexual behavior, as are some Western cultures today. By the same token gay and bisexual behavior has become an entrenched though hidden part of very intolerant institutions such as armies and prisons. The oppression of homo- and bisexuality can lead to both physical and psychological violence. Indeed many oppressed gays and bisexuals fight back by oppressing others. Only tolerant approaches to sexuality can break the chain of oppression from generation to generation.

THE DREAM DILEMMA

People cannot live without dreams about their future. But some dreams can prevent others from being realized. The social dream of democracy keeps many from seeing how truly undemocratic society can be. Homo- and bisexuality are imagined by many to be a traducer of their dream of a homogeneous, heterosexual heaven on earth. In a kind of self-fulfilling prophecy, behavior looked on by the majority as deviant and unnatural forces those who practice it to go underground. Thus the majority does not see the internalized oppression occurring. What they will see are unexplainable suicides, sexual crimes, blackmail, disappearances, robberies, and violence not reported to the police. And when some of this comes to the surface, it will only "prove" the necessity to oppress the sexual preference considered to be the "cause" of all this misery. But in fact it is society's incapacity to give shape and meaning to individual self-determination that is doing the harm.

This does not mean that social dreams are dangerous in general. People need to believe in and follow their dreams. But as soon as people derive the right to impose their views upon others from that dream, human rights are endangered. The democratic quality of a society can only be measured by the degree to which it accepts the right of individual self-determination.

THE PROHIBITION PARADOX

Alcohol, drugs, sex, and prostitution are ideal examples of the prohibition paradox: by outlawing acts among consenting adults one does not prevent but creates criminality. Each legal system that neglects the right to individual self-determination creates problems it cannot solve, not even by reshaping society into one huge prison. Bans on alcohol did not prevent its consumption but only stimulated crime. In countries where the use of drugs is legal under certain conditions (as in the Netherlands) the use is declining, whereas drug use is rising in those countries trying to forbid it completely.

Anti-homosexual legislation never has been effective in stopping homosexual behavior; instead it has led to suicides, blackmail, and security risks. Neither homosexuality nor bisexuality in itself creates a security risk. The prohibition of it does. The exploitation of people is the real problem, not their sexual behavior. The legalization of prostitution proves this: prostitutes are more exploited in countries which made prostitution illegal than in countries with safeguards for the right to self-determination of sex workers.

REDEFINING REALITIES

Many people assume that our lives are determined by powers mightier than ourselves—perhaps Nature, Society, God, or Science. Such belief can, again, create a self-fulfilling prophecy: by defining a situation as real, we can make it real in its consequences. But we cannot change all situations just by redefining them. While there are many examples of the importance of defining situations—one of the most important tasks for social scientists being to investigate the possibility for changing existing living situations—it is useless to invest time and energy trying to change situations that cannot be changed.

A situation's potential for change depends on the conditions under which change can take place. First, people must be aware of the fact that things have been and can be changed. Here, intercultural comparisons are very important. When we all live in the same way (or assume we do), it is very difficult to imagine alternative lifestyles. That is one of the reasons why the acceptance of pluralism is so important for the survival of culture. Without pluralism, cultures will die. Most people think uniformity is a symbol of strength, but in fact it is the opposite. Only well-integrated societies can afford multiformity. Weaker cultures or societies underestimating their strength tend to look for solutions in a counterproductive way. In many cases we construct determinations ourselves and thus become victims of avoidable acts that we ourselves are responsible for.

By persecuting feelings that damage nobody, we create monsters that might destroy us. By making homo- and bisexuality illegal, and by trying to prevent gays, lesbians, and bisexuals from entering the army or secret services, states did create security risks where they could have been avoided by not discriminating against homo- and bisexuals. This is one of the reasons why some governments do not discriminate any more against gays and lesbians in the police, army, and foreign and secret services. No one can blackmail an openly gay or bisexual person with his or her sexual orientation.

In the past, left-handed people were discriminated against because people thought that left-handedness was a sign of deviancy or the mark of the devil. Fortunately, people became aware that it was not left-handedness in itself that was a problem but the societal discrimination against it. Similarly, homosexuality does not harm anybody but it nevertheless became labeled as a sin, disease, or deviance. The growing respect for human rights and its underlying principle of individual self-determination stimulated an increasing tolerance of and respect for different sexual lifestyles. Those who continue to discriminate against gays and bisexuals are not only endangering these groups but also their own right to self-determination.

EDUCATION EFFORTS

How can AIDS information and education slow down the spread of HIV among bisexuals and their partners? Thanks to the WHO, an inventory has been made of the most effective AIDS information and education campaigns from various countries. Attention was focused on the extent to which these campaigns managed to reach gays and bisexuals, and their possible impact upon the sexual lifestyles of both these groups. An analysis of those campaigns makes clear that they have the following characteristics in common.

The use of *community-based prevention models* seems to be of utmost importance. Those campaigns stressing community involvement help in developing prevention activities by increasing the level of commitment of people at risk who now consider the prevention message as their own instead of somebody else's. Such community development among bisexuals is vital for effective AIDS prevention efforts.

On a national level, the *development of AIDS prevention programs* is essential. Their efficacy increases when their work is based upon the human-rights principles of individual self-determination, equal treatment, privacy, informed consent, and access to employment, social security, housing, and health care. By doing so, they create an atmosphere of justice, shared responsibility, and common effort, and they avoid unnecessary tensions and conflicts. But by neglecting the specific aspects of bisexuality and AIDS, these same programs harm not only the welfare of men who engage in bisexual contacts but society at large.

Many campaigns are presenting moralistic (often anti-sexual) views. The problem is that moralistic campaigns tend to be counterproductive in reaching people at risk. People are often inclined to ignore views which they perceive as being imposed upon them. *Fact-oriented nonmoralistic campaigns* are therefore more likely to stimulate less risky behavior. This applies even more to sensitive topics like bisexuality and AIDS. It is important to develop differentiated messages adapted to specific target groups, but the content of the messages should be the same.

The development of prevention campaigns by organizations representing people of the target group involved, and the evaluation by researchers trusted by them, are *creating effective feedback mechanisms.* This enables policy makers to react quickly to trends in attitudes and behavior in the groups to be reached. Otherwise campaign planners would be acting like captains on a ship without any knowledge about the sea they are sailing on. Feedback on more closeted risk groups is complicated but not impossible, as some authors in this book have described.

Using *sexually explicit language* instead of vague and ambiguous terms such as "exchange of body fluids" might be difficult in many societies. However, unnecessary panic can be avoided by doing so. One can be explicit without being offensive. The notion that the mere mention of bisexual behavior might be too explosive even to be mentioned in educational materials could result in many needless deaths and should therefore not be acceptable in an effective AIDS campaign. On the other hand, it is important to *avoid judgmental terms* like "drug abuse" (instead of drug use), "risk groups" (instead of risky behavior), "promiscuous sex" (instead of risky sex), "innocent victims" (instead of people infected), and "homos" (instead of men having sex with men). The use of judgmental terms makes it easier for people to think they themselves are not involved. By focusing campaigns on concrete behavior, it is more difficult for everyone to ignore the message. Bisexual men specifically are extremely sensitive to judgmental language. These sensitivities can be alleviated by focusing on factual descriptions of behavior instead of identity-related judgments.

Campaigns must emphasize the fact that the virus is *transmitted*

by human activities, not by groups or places. As long as HIV transmission is identified with groups or places, people tend to feel safe by
avoiding them while continuing unsafe activities. By doing so, the spread
of HIV is in fact stimulated. Moreover, focusing on groups and places
creates all kinds of stigmatization and discrimination, which has a negative
effect on the efficacy of the prevention activities. By saying that "bisexuals
are the bridge between the infected gay community and the rest of society,"
one tends to forget that everybody is a potential bridge as long as we
are involved in risky behavior. We should not blame a specific group
for a responsibility to be shared by everybody.

By *highlighting the shared responsibility of both infector and infected
for transmitting the virus,* everybody will accept the responsibility of
avoiding risky behavior. If campaigns only focus on people with HIV/
AIDS to act safely, situations are created in which people are tempted
to hide their status and infect others. If everybody is acting in a safe
way, the irresponsible behavior of potential infectors will not result in
new infections because of the precautions being taken by others. The
education policy of shared responsibility is therefore much more effective
than policies which give some people the impression that they are less
responsible for the spread of the virus than others. Bisexual men are
as responsible as everybody else for protecting themselves and others
against avoidable risks.

By *avoiding stigmatization and discrimination* of people involved,
prevention campaigns make it easier to develop cooperation with those
whom they want to reach. For instance: by connecting homo- and
bisexuality with the image of AIDS, the general public often assumes
that AIDS has nothing to do with them, and gay or bisexual communities feel discriminated against. By focusing on specific sexual techniques
involving risk, everybody practicing those techniques can be reached
regardless of his or her sexual identification. Specific prevention activities by bisexual men would remain necessary, but should not be limited
to them alone. That is why more attention has to be paid to bisexuality
as another form of sexual behavior, especially in those countries where
it has been a taboo subject up to now.

Preventing hysteria provoked by mass media is essential in good
prevention campaigns. Hysteria and panic produce shock effects for
only very short periods of time. In the long run they are counterproductive because they tend to make people insensitive to real risks. By offering expert support to journalists, the quality of the media reporting
on AIDS can be improved. Bisexuality is in many countries a source

of sensationalist media attention. Our efforts should be not to ignore or to exaggerate bisexuality but to enlighten everybody about the realities of life, including our sexual life.

By *offering opportunities for anonymous and individual information,* the efficacy of AIDS education can be increased dramatically. General prevention messages tend to cause all kinds of misunderstanding. By being able to communicate with an individual, even the most secret fears and behaviors can be discussed. AIDS hotlines and AIDS counseling services, in addition to general prevention activities, can therefore be very helpful in reaching those people difficult to reach. This is specifically true for bisexual men and their partners.

By *supporting the self-organization of people at risk,* prevention policy makers enable themselves to communicate more effectively with the people they want to reach. Those countries that support the gay and bisexual emancipation movement, organizations of injecting drug users, prostitutes and their clients, and people with HIV and/or AIDS have been more successful in developing effective prevention strategies among those at risk. This kind of support does not necessarily mean that we condone the behaviors referred to above, but that we accept the shared responsibility in order to create a society based upon the principle of self-determination.

The *production and distribution of free information on AIDS* have been very effective, especially when combined with STD prevention and condom promotion activities. The spread of STDs is an important indicator of risky sexual behavior. Therefore, AIDS and STD-prevention campaigns need to complement each other. The same applies to drug-prevention campaigns, and methadon and needle exchange programs: free, nonjudgmental, and reliable information combined with possibilities for personal guidance are evaluated positively by those involved.

Free and anonymous HIV-testing facilities, combined with prevention information, have been very effective in many countries in making people aware of the risks they have been exposed to. The testing itself is not a guarantee of future safe behavior. Personal guidance before, during, and after testing is of the utmost importance. Counselor training is necessary, with specific attention being paid to homo- and bisexuality.

The World Health Organization plays an important role in stimulating AIDS research. According to WHO standards, researchers accept the *informed consent principle in AIDS research*: all participants are informed about the goals of the research and left free either to stay with or to leave the project. Prevention-oriented research has enabled us to analyze the effects of AIDS information and education activities. Participants in this and similar research projects have the right to receive feedback on their own behavior if they wish.

The acceptance of the privacy principle in the sensitive research surrounding AIDS is essential. Anonymity of the respondents has to be guaranteed, and the confidentiality of the relation between researcher and respondents deserves necessary minimum safeguards. This is not only in the interest of the participating individuals but also to enhance the reliability of the research. Many countries do not have research findings regarding risky behavior in their society, which makes it very difficult for prevention policy makers to assess the real needs of AIDS information and education campaigns.

The acceptance of social and ethical guidelines by interdisciplinary advice committees to guide prevention and research has been important in preventing societal conflicts over ethically sensitive issues. The human rights declarations, based upon the individual's right to self-determination, create a solid basis for socially and ethically responsible AIDS education activities.

By *international cooperation* we can learn from each other: we do not need to reinvent the wheel in every country. Although each culture has its own specific cultural characteristics, we can nevertheless learn from each other's experiences to prevent the spread of the virus by recognizing common mechanisms in human behavior. By focusing on prevention intentions and ignoring factual results, some education campaigns can be counterproductive. By focusing on factual prevention effects, AIDS education can be very effective in slowing the spread of the virus. In fact, in some countries, AIDS education campaigns have been more effective than most health education programs in the past.

RELEVANT RESEARCH

This volume on bisexuality and HIV/AIDS demonstrates that there is an urgent need for more information on sexual behavior of bisexual men as well as their sexual partners. In most countries people are unaware of the potential risk of spreading HIV/AIDS by bisexual contacts. Cross-cultural research is needed to describe and analyze the mechanisms of bisexual behavior and its consequences for future development of the AIDS epidemic. That is why an international network of psychosocial researchers since 1989 has started to investigate, by qualitative and quantitative methods, the various aspects of bisexuality and HIV/AIDS. This project is sponsored by the World Health Organization/Global Programme on AIDS and the government of the Netherlands, and is coordinated by the Gay and Lesbian Studies Department of the University of Utrecht.

Mailing Address:
Gay and Lesbian Studies Department
University of Utrecht
P.O. Box 80140
NL–3508 TC Utrecht
The Netherlands

References

Abrams, D.; C. Abraham; R. Spears; and D. Marks. 1990. "AIDS In-vulnerability: Relationships, Sexual Behavior, and Attitudes Among 16–19-Year-Olds." In P. Aggleton, D. Davies, and H. Hart, eds. *AIDS: Individual, Cultural, and Policy Dimensions*. London: Falmer.

AIDS Coordination Team of the Netherlands. 1987. *AIDS Information and Education: A Policy Report*.

Ajzen, I., and M. Fishbein. 1980. *Understanding Attitudes and Predicting Social Behavior*. Englewood Cliffs, N.J.: Prentice-Hall.

Allen, D. M. 1980. "Young Male Prostitutes: A Psychosocial Study." *Archives of Sexual Behavior* 9 (5): 399–427.

Anonymous. 1989. Personal experience reported in a Thai gay magazine. *Morakot* 4 (37): 94.

————. 1990. Personal experience reported in a Thai gay magazine. *Neon*, No. 52: 110–11.

Arnold, W., and F. Barnes. 1989. "Peer Education Program Reaches High-Risk Adolescents with AIDS Information and Prevention." Paper presented at the Fifth International Conference on AIDS, Montreal.

Ary, R. M. 1987. *Gay: Dunia ganjil kaum homofil* [Gay: Homophiles' Odd World]. Jakarta: Grafiti.

Atmojo, Kemala. 1987. [1986]. *Kami bukan lekaki* [*We Are Not Men*]. Jakarta: Grafiti.

Bakeman, R.; J. R. Lumb; R. Jackson; and D. W. Smith. 1986. "AIDS Statistics and the Risk for Minorities." *AIDS Research* 2: 249–52.

————; E. McCray; J. R. Lumb; R. E. Jackson; and P. N. Whitley. 1987. "The Incidence of AIDS Among Blacks and Hispanics." *Journal of The National Medical Association* 78: 921–28.

Bancroft, J. 1983. *Human Sexuality and Its Problems*. London: Churchill-Livingstone.

Bandura, M. H. 1977. "Self-Efficacy: Toward a Unifying Theory of Behavioral Change. *Psychological Review* 84: 191–215.

———. 1982. "Self-Efficacy Mechanism in Human Agency." *American Psychologist* 37: 122–47.

Banerjea, J. H. 1956. "Cult Syncretism," Vol. 4 of *The Cultural Heritage of India*. Calcutta: Ramakrishna Mission Institute of Culture.

Barr, E. 1985. "Chicago Bi-Ways: An Informal History." In *Bisexualities: Theory and Research*, F. Klein and T. Wolf, eds. New York: Haworth Press.

Battjes, R. J.; R. W. Pickens; and Z. Amsel. 1989. "Introduction of HIV Infection Among Intravenous Drug Abusers in Low Prevalence Areas." *Journal of Acquired Immune Deficiency Syndrome* 2: 533–39.

Beach, R. S., et al. 1989. "HIV Infection in Brazil." *New England Journal of Medicine* 321:830.

Becker, M. H. 1974. "The Health Belief Model and Personal Health Behavior." *Health Education Monographs* 2: 220–43.

———, and J. G. Joseph. 1988. "AIDS and Behavioral Change to Reduce Risk: A Review." *American Journal of Public Health* 78: 394–410.

Bell, A., and M. Weinberg. 1978. *Homosexualities: A Study of Diversity Among Men and Women*. New York: Simon & Schuster.

Bennett, G.; S. Chapman; and F. Bray. 1989a. "Sexual Practices and 'Beats': AIDS-Related Sexual Practices in a Sample of Homosexual and Bisexual Men in the Western Area of Sydney." *Medical Journal of Australia* 151: 306–14.

———. 1989b. "A Potential Source for the Transmission of the Human Immuno-deficiency Virus into the Heterosexual Population: Bisexual Men Who Frequent 'Beats'." *Medical Journal of Australia* 151: 314–18.

Berg, D. L., and J. Berg. 1988. "AIDS in Prison: The Social Construction of a Reality." *International Journal of Offender Therapy & Comparative Criminology* 2: 17–28.

Bergamaschi, D., et al. 1989. "Pediatric AIDS in Brazil: Description and Analysis of Trends." Paper presented at the Fifth International Conference on AIDS, Montreal.

Bhattacharya, S. 1978. *The Indian Theogony*, Firma. Calcutta: KLM Pvt. Ltd.

Bloor, M.; N. McKeganey; and M. Barnard. 1990. "An Ethnographic Study of HIV-Related Risk Practices Among Glasgow Rent Boys and Their Clients: Report of a Pilot Study." *AIDS Care* 2: 17–24.

Blumstein, P. W., and P. Schwartz. 1977. "Bisexuality: Some Sociological Issues." *Journal of Social Issues* 2: 30–45.

Boles, J.; M. Sweat; and A. Elifson. 1989. "Bisexuality Among Male Prostitutes." Paper presented at the CDC Workshop on Bisexuality and AIDS, Atlanta, Ga.

Bouhdiba, A. 1975. *Sexuality in Islam*. London: Routledge & Kegan Paul.

Boulton, M.; Z. Schramm Evans; R. Fitzpatrick; and G. Hart. 1989. "Bisexual Men: Identity and Behavior in Sexual Encounters." Paper presented at the Twenty-First Annual Conference of the Medical Sociology Group, Manchester, England.

Boyer, D. 1989. "Male Prostitution and Homosexual Identity." *Journal of Homosexuality* 17 (1 and 2): 151–84.

Bradford, N. 1983. "Transgenderism and the Cult of Yellamma: Heat, Sex, and Sickness in South Indian Ritual." *Journal of Anthropological Research* 39: 307–22.

Branden, P. 1990–. Ongoing study of sexual practices of Family Planning Clinic patients in Christchurch, New Zealand.

Brandes, S. 1981. "Like Wounded Stags: Male Sexual Ideology in an Andalusian Town." In *Sexual Meanings*, H. Whitehead and S. Ortner, eds. London: Cambridge University Press.

Brandt, A. M. 1988. "AIDS in Historical Perspective: Four Lessons from the History of Sexually Transmitted Diseases." *American Journal of Public Health* 78: 367–71.

Budiman, Amen. 1979. *Lelaki perindu lelaki* [*Men Who Long for Men*]. Semarang: Tanjung Sari.

Bunnag, P. 1990a. "Wanting to Be the Officer's Lady." *Midway* (a Thai gay magazine) 2 (27): 12–14.

———. 1990b. "Gay Video Saved a Marriage." *Midway* 2 (28): 73–74.

———. 1990c. "When a Man Becomes a Woman." *Midway* 2 (27): 47–48.

Burke, R., and T. Weir. 1982. "Husband-Wife Helping Relationships as Moderators of Experienced Stress: The 'Mental Hygiene' Function in Marriage." In *Family Stress, Coping, and Social Support*, H. McCubbin, A. Cauble, and J. Patterson, eds. Springfield, Ill.: Charles Thomas.

Butts, W. H. 1947. "Boy Prostitutes in the Metropolis." *Journal of Clinical Psychopathology* 8: 673–81.

Callendar, J. M., and L. M. Kochems. 1983. "The North American Berdache." *Current Anthropology* 24:443–56.
———. 1986. "Men and Not-Men: Male Gender-Mixing Statuses and Homosexuality." *Journal of Homosexuality* 11 (3 and 4): 5–78.
Came, H. 1988. "What Are the Implications of Heterosexism and Homosexism to Bisexuals?" Unpublished manuscript.
Caplan, G. 1964. *Principles of Preventive Psychiatry*. New York: Basic Books.
Caplan, P., ed. 1987. *The Cultural Construction of Sexuality*. London: Tavistock Press.
Carael, M., and P. Piot. 1989. "HIV Infection in Developing Countries." *Journal of Biosociology* 10 (supp.): 35–50.
Carballo-Diéguez, A. 1989. "Hispanic Culture, Gay Male Culture, and AIDS.: Counseling Implications." *Journal of Counseling and Development* 68: 26–30.
Cargill, V. A. 1989. "SAMM—Stopping AIDS Is My Mission: A Minority Adolescent AIDS Education Program." Paper presented at the Fifth International Conference on AIDS, Montreal.
Carrier, J. M. 1971. "Participants in Urban Male Homosexual Encounters." *Archives of Sexual Behavior* 1 (4): 79–91.
———. 1976. "Cultural Factors Affecting Urban Mexican Male Homosexual Encounters." *Archives of Sexual Behavior* 5: 103–24.
———. 1985. "Mexican Male Bisexuality." In *Bisexualities: Theory and Research*, F. Klein and J. Wolf, eds. New York: Haworth Press, pp. 75–85.
———. 1988. "Gay Liberation and Coming Out in Mexico." *Journal of Homosexuality* 17: 225–52.
———. 1989. "Sexual Behavior and the Spread of AIDS in Mexico." *Medical Anthropology Quarterly* 10 (2 and 3): 129–42.
———, and J. R. Magaña. N.d. "Applied Anthropology and AIDS in a Health Care Agency." Unpublished manuscript.
Castilho, E., et al. 1989. "Patterns and Trends of Heterosexual Transmission of HIV Among Brazilan AIDS Cases." Paper presented at the Fifth International Conference on AIDS, Montreal.
Catania, J. A.; S. M. Kegeles; and T. J. Coates. 1990. "Towards an Understanding of Risk Behavior: An AIDS Risk-Reduction Model (ARRM)." *Health Education Quarterly*.

Caukins, N. R. 1974. "Male Prostitution: A Psychosocial View of Behavior.," *American Journal of Orthopsychiatry* 44: 782–85.

Caukins, S. E., and N. R. Coombs. 1976. "The Psychodynamics of Male Prostitution." *The American Journal of Psychotherapy*: 441–51.

Centers for Disease Control. 1986. "Acquired Immunodeficiency Syndrome (AIDS) Among Blacks and Hispanics—United States." *MMWR* 15: 655–58; 663–66.

———. 1989a. "HIV/AIDS Surveillance." U.S. Department of Services.

———. 1989b. "Update: Heterosexual Transmission of Acquired Immunodeficiency Syndrome and Human Immunodeficiency Virus Infection—United States." *MMWR* 38: 423–34.

Centers for Disease Control. 1990. *HIV/AIDS Surveillance Report*. Atlanta. Centers for Disease Control.

Chetwynd, J. 1989. "A Case Study of the Burnett Clinic." Part of WHO Program in AIDS counseling case studies.

———, and T. Hughes. 1990. "Characteristics of Those Attending the Burnett Clinic for Pre- and Post-HIV Test Counseling."

Chetwynd, S. J. 1987. *A National Survey of NZ Attitudes, Knowledge, and Behavior Relating to AIDS*. Wellington, New Zealand.

Chin, J., and J. Mann. 1990. "HIV Infections and AIDS in the 1990s." *Annual Review of Public Health* 11.

Christophersen, J., et al. 1988. "Sexually Transmitted Diseases in Hetero-, Homo-, and Bisexual Males in Copenhagen." *Danish Medical Bulletin* 35 (3): 285–88.

Chu, S. V.; L. S. Doll; and J. W. Buehler. 1989. "Epidemiology of AIDS in Bisexual Males."

Coggeshall, J. M. 1988. "Ladies Behind Bars: A Liminal Gender as Cultural Mirror." *Anthropology Today* 4: 6–9.

Chompootaweep, S., et al. 1988. *A Study of Reproductive Health in Adolescence of Secondary School Students and Teachers in Bangkok*. Chulangkorn University: Institute of Health Research.

Coleman, E. 1987. "Assessment of Sexual Orientation." *Journal of Homosexuality* 14: 9–24.

———. 1988. "The Development of Male Prostitution Activity Among Gay and Bisexual Adolescents." *Journal of Homosexuality* 17: 131–49.

Collaborative Study Group. 1989. "HIV Infection in Patients Attending Clinics for Sexually Transmitted Diseases in England and Wales." *British Medical Journal* 298: 415–18.

Connell, R., et al. 1989. "Unsafe Anal Sexual Practice Among Homosexual and Bisexual Men." *Social Aspects of the Prevention of AIDS Study: Report No. 6.* Macquarrie University.

Cortes, E., et al. 1989. "HIV-1, HIV-2, and HTLV-1 Infection in High-Risk Groups in Brazil." *New England Journal of Medicine* 320 (15): 953–58.

Coughlin, T. A. 1988. "AIDS in Prison: One Correctional Administrator's Recomended Policies and Procedures." *Judicature* 72(1); 63–70.

Coutinho, R. A.; R. L. Van Andel; and T. S. Rijsdijk. 1988. "Role of Male Prostitutes in the Spread of Sexually Transmitted Diseases and HIV." *Genito-Urinary Medicine* 64 (3): 207–208.

Creed, G. W. 1984. "Sexual Subordination: Institutionalized Homosexuality and Social Control in Melanesia." *Ethnology* 23: 157–76.

Dandekar, R. N. 1962. *Indian Mythology in the Cultural Heritage of India.* Calcutta: Ramakrishna Mission Institute of Culture.

Davenport, W. 1977. "Sex in Cross-Cultural Perspective." In *Human Sexuality in Four Perspectives*, F. A. Beach and M. Diamond, eds. Baltimore, Md.: Johns Hopkins University Press.

Davies, P.; A. Hunt; M. Macourt; and P. Weatherburn. 1990. "Longitudinal Study of Sexual Behavior of Homosexually Active Males under the Impact of AIDS." *Project Sigma: Final Report to the Department of Health.*

Day, S. 1988. "Prostitute Women with AIDS: Anthropology" (editorial review). *AIDS* 2: 421–28.

De la Vega, E. 1989. "Homosexuality and Bisexuality Among Latino Men." *Focus* (June): 3–4.

———. N.d. "Observations on Bisexual Behavior within the U.S. Latino Context." Unpublished manuscript.

Department of Health. 1989. *Update of the 1987 Survey of KABP Relating to AIDS.* Wellington, New Zealand.

Devi, S. 1977. *The World of Homosexuals.* New Delhi: Vikas.

DiClemente, R.; L. Zorn; and L. Temoshok. 1986. "Adolescents and AIDS: A Survey of Knowledge, Attitude, and Beliefs about AIDS in San Francisco." *American Journal of Public Health* 76: 1443–45.

Dirección General de Epidemiología. 1990. Situación del SIDA en México, hasta el 30 de Marzo de 1990." *Boletín Mensual* 4: 844–53.

Division of AIDS. 1990. *AIDS Newsletter* (November). Ministry of Public Health: Department of Communicable Disease Control.

Division of Epidemiology. 1990. *Results from the First, Second, and Third Rounds of the Sentinel Surveillance System on HIV, June 1989, December 1989, and June 1990.* Bangkok, Thailand.

Doll, L. S., et al. 1990a. "Factors Relating to the Persistence of High-Risk Sexual Behavior Among Homosexuals: A Multi-Center Comparison." Unpublished manuscript.

——, and HIV Donor Study Group. 1990b. "Homosexually and Non-homosexually Identified Male Blood Donors Who Have Sex With Men: A Behavioral Comparison." Abstract submitted to the Sixth Annual Conference on AIDS, San Francisco.

——; L. Peterson; C. W. White; and HIV Blood Donor Study Group. 1990c. "HIV-1 Seropositive Blood Donors: A Multi-Center Analysis of Who They Are and Why They Donate Blood." Unpublished manuscript.

Donoghoe, M. C.; G. V. Stimson; K. Dolan; and L. Alldritt. 1989. "Changes in HIV Risk Behavior in Clients of Syringe-Exchange Schemes in England and Scotland." *AIDS* 3: 267–72.

Donovan, J. E., and R. Jessor. 1985. "Structure of Problem-Solving Behavior in Adolescence and Young Adulthood." *Journal of Consulting and Clinical Psychology* 53: 890–904.

Dover, K. J. 1978. *Greek Homosexuality.* New York: Vintage.

Eckstrand, M. 1989. "Prevalence and Change in High-Risk Sexual Behaviors Among Bisexual Men in San Francisco." Paper presented at the CDC Workshop on Bisexuality and AIDS, Atlanta, Ga.

——, and T. J. Coates. 1990. "Gay Men in San Francisco Are Maintaining Low-Risk Behaviors But Young Men Continue to Be at Risk." *American Journal of Public Health.*

——; T. J. Coates; S. Lang; and J. Guydish. 1989. "Prevalence and Change of AIDS High-Risk Sexual Behavior Among Bisexual Men in San Francisco." The San Francisco Men's Health Study Abstracts from the Fifth International Conference on AIDS, Montreal.

Elifson, K. W., et al. 1989. "Seroprevalence of Human Immunodeficiency Virus Among Male Prostitutes." *New England Journal of Medicine* 321: 822–33.

Ellenberger, H. F. 1970. *The Discovery of the Unconscious. The History and Evolution of Dynamic Psychiatry.* London: Allen Lane.

Emmons, C. A., et al. 1987. "Psychosocial Predictors of Reported Behavior Change in Homosexual Men at Risk of AIDS." *Health Education Quarterly* 13: 31–45.

European Study Group.1989. "Rise Factors for Male to Female Transmission of HIV." *British Medical Journal* 298: 215–18.

Evans, B., et al. 1989. "Trends in Sexual Behavior and Risk Factors for HIV Infection Among Homosexual Men." *Genito-Urinary Medicine* 65: 259–62.

Evans-Pritchard, E. E. 1974. *Man and Woman Among the Azande.* London: Faber and Faber.

Farah, M. 1984. *Marriage and Sexuality in Islam.* Salt Lake City: University of Utah Press.

Fay, R. E.; C. F. Turner; A. D. Klassen; and J. H. Gagnon. 1989. "Prevalence and Patterns of Same-Gender Sexual Contact Among Men." *Science* 243 (4889): 338–48.

Feldman, D. A. 1986. "Anthropology, AIDS, and Africa." *Medical Anthropology Quarterly* 17 (2): 38–40.

———. 1988. "Gay Youths and AIDS." *Journal of Homosexuality* 17: 185–93.

Fishbein, M. 1980. "A Theory of Reasoned Action: Some Applications and Implications." In *Nebraska Symposium on Motivation, 1979,* H. E. Howe and M. M. Page, eds. Reading, Me.: Addison-Wesley.

———, and I. Ajzen. 1975. *Belief, Attitude, Intention, and Behavior: An Introduction to Theory and Research.* Reading, Me.: Addison-Wesley.

Fisher, B.; K. Weisberg; and T. Marotta. 1982. *Report on Adolescent Male Prostitution.* San Francisco: Urban & Rural Systems Associates.

Fitzpatrick, R., et al. 1989. "Heterosexual Sexual Behavior in a Sample of Homosexually Active Men." *Genito-Urinary Medicine* 65: 259–62.

———; M. Boulton; and G. Hart. 1990. *Health Beliefs and Health Behavior to Male Homosexuals in Relation to AIDS: Final Report to the Medical Research Council.*

Ford, C. S., and F. A. Beach. 1952. *Patterns of Sexual Behavior.* London: Byre & Spottiswoode.

Forman, D., and C. Chilvers. 1989. "Sexual Behavior of Young and Middle-Aged Men in England and Wales." *British Medical Journal* 298: 1137–42.

Freud, S. 1905, 1961. *Three Essays on the Theory of Sexuality.* Vol. 7 of *The Standard Edition of the Complete Works of Sigmund Freud,* J. Strachey, ed. and trans. London: Hogarth Press.

Freud, S. 1925. *Some Psychical Consequences of the Anatomical Distinction between the Sexes.* Vol. 19 of *The Standard Edition of the Complete Works of Sigmund Freud*, J. Strachey, ed. and trans. London: Hogarth Press.

Freund, K.; H. Scher; S. Chan; and M. Ben-Aron. 1982. "Experimental Analysis of Pedophilia." *Behavioral Research and Therapy* 20: 105–12.

Fry, P. 1982. *Para ingles ver.* Rio de Janeiro. Zahar Editores.

————. 1985. "Male Homosexuality and Spirit Possession in Brazil." *Journal of Homosexuality* 11 (3 and 4): 137–53.

————, and E. MacRae. 1983. *O que é homossexualidade.* São Paulo: Editora Brasiliense.

Gagnon, J. H. 1977. *Human Sexualities.* Glenview, Ill.: Scott, Foresman.

————. 1989. "The Management of Erotic Relations with Both Genders." Paper presented at the CDC Workshop on Bisexuality and AIDS, Atlanta, Ga.

————. 1989. "Disease and Desire." *Daedalus* 118 (3): 46–77.

————, and W. Simon. 1977. *Sexual Conduct.* Chicago: Aldens Publishing Co.

Gallo-Silver, A., et al. 1989. "Psycho-Social Issues Presented by Self-Identified Bisexual Men with HIV Conditions." Abstract of a paper presented at the Fifth International Conference on AIDS, Montreal.

García, M. L., et al. 1989. "Male Bisexuality and AIDS, Present Status and Perspective in Mexico." Paper presented at the Fifth International Conference on AIDS, Montreal.

Gerstel, C. J.; A. J. Feraios, and G. Herdt. 1989. "Widening Circles: An Ethnographic Profile of a Youth Group." *Journal of Homosexuality* 17: 75–92.

Gibson, P. 1988. "The Risk of AIDS in Young Gay and Bisexual Males." *Focus* 12: 3–4.

Ginsburg, K. N. 1967. "The 'Meat Rack': A Study of the Male Homosexual Prostitute." *American Journal of Psychotherapy* 21: 170–85.

Gluckman, L. K. 1974. "Transcultural Considerations of Homosexuality with Special Reference to the NZ Maori. *Australian-New Zealand Journal of Psychiatry* 8: 121–25.

Gochros, J. 1982. "When Husbands Come Out of the Closet: A Study on the Consequences for Their Wives." Diss. University of Denver. *UMI Abstracts* 8315, 899.

Gochros, J. 1989. *When Husbands Come Out of the Closet.* New York: Haworth Press.

Gray, P. 1986. "Growing Yams and Men: An Interpretation of Kiman Male Ritualized Homosexual Behavior." *Journal of Homosexuality* 11 (3 and 4): 55–56.

Griggs, T., et al. 1989. "The Development of a Street-Based Outreach Program to Reach Young Male, Female, and Transsexual Street-Based Prostitutes in Sydney, Australia." Paper presented at the Fifth International Conference on AIDS, Montreal.

Hansen, C. E., and A. Evans. 1985. "Bisexuality Reconsidered: An Idea in Pursuit of a Definition." *Journal of Homosexuality* 11 (1 and 2): 1–6.

Hanson, H., ed. 1990. *Bisexuele levens in Nederland.* Amsterdam: Orlando.

Hays, D., and A. Samuels. 1989. "Heterosexual Women's Perceptions of Their Marriages to Bisexual or Homosexual Men." *Journal of Homosexuality* 18: 81–100.

———; S. M. Kegeles; and T. J. Coates. "High HIV Risk-Taking Among Young Gay Men. AIDS." In press.

Heilbrun, C. 1973. *Towards a Recognition of Androgyny.* New York: Knopf.

Herdt, G. H. 1981. *Guardians of the Flutes: Idioms of Masculinity.* New York: McGraw-Hill.

Herdt, G. H. 1982. "Fetish and Fantasy in Sambian Initiation." In *Ritual of Manhood: Male Initiation in New Guinea,* G. Herdt, ed. Berkeley: University of California Press.

———, ed. 1984. *Ritualized Homosexuality in Melanesia.* Berkeley: University of California Press.

———. 1985. "A Comment on Cultural Attributes and Fluidity of Bisexuality." *Journal of Homosexuality* 10: 53–61.

———. 1988. "Introduction: Gay and Lesbian Youth, Emergent Identities, and Cultural Scenes at Home and Abroad." *Journal of Homosexuality* 17: 1–41.

———. 1989. "Bisexuality in Cultural Context." Paper presented at the CDC Workshop on Bisexuality and AIDS, Atlanta, Ga.

Hill, L., and C. Crothers. 1988. *The Literature on New Zealand Sexuality.* University of Auckland.

HIV/AIDS Surveillance Monthly Reports. Atlanta, Ga.: Centers for Disease Control.

Horne, J.; J. Chetwynd; and J. Kelleher. 1989. *Changing Sexual Practices Among Homosexual Men in Response to AIDS: Who Has Changed, Who Hasn't, and Why?* Wellington, New Zealand: Report to the Department of Health.

Hospedales, C. J., and S. Mahibir. 1988. "The Epidemiology of AIDS in the Caribbean and Action to Date." In *The Global Impact of AIDS*, Alan Fleming et al., eds. Pp. 27–33. New York: Alan R. Liss, Inc.

Hrdy, D. B. 1987. "Cultural Practices Contributing to the Transmission of Human Immuno-Deficiency Virus in Africa." *Review of Infectious Diseases* 10 (6): 1106–19.

Humphreys, R. A. L. 1970. *Tearoom Trade: A Study of Homosexual Encounters in Public Places.* London: Duckworth.

———. 1975. *Tearoom Trade: Impersonal Sex in Public Places.* Chicago: Aldine Press.

Irwin, J. 1980. *Prisons in Turmoil.* Boston: Little Brown and Company.

Izazola, J. A.; L. Pineda; J. L. Valdespino; and J. Sepúlveda. 1989. "Condom Use and Knowledge in General Population, Female Prostitutes and Gay and Bisexual Men." Paper presented at the Fifth International Conference on AIDS, Montreal.

Janis, I. L. 1967. "Effects of Fear Arousal on Attitude Change: Recent Developments in Theory and Research." Vol. 3 of *Advances in Experimental Social Psychology*, L. Berkowitz, ed. New York: Academic Press.

Janz, N. K., and M. H. Becker. 1984. "The Health Belief Model: A Decade Later." *Health Education Quarterly* 11: 1–47.

Jeyasingh, P.; S. D. Fernandes; V. Ganesan; and T. B. Ramanaiah. 1986. "A Study of Use of Condoms by Men Attending STD Clinics." *Indian Journal of Sexually Transmitted Disease* 7: 27–29.

Johnson, L. D.; P. M. O'Malley; and J. G. Bavchman. 1985. *Use of Licit and Illicit Drugs by America's High School Students, 1975–1984.* U.S. Department of Health and Human Services. DHHS Publications No. (ADM) 85–1384.

Jones, C., and D. Vlahov,. 1990. "Why Don't Intravenous Drug Users Use Condoms?" *Journal of Acquired Immune Deficiency Syndrome* 2: 416–417.

Joseph, J., et al. 1987. "Perceived Risk of AIDS: Assessing the Behavioral and Psychsocial Consequences in a Cohort of Gay Men." *Journal of Applied Social Psychology* 17: 231–50.

Joshi, U. V.; S. O. Cameron; J. M. Sommerville; and R. G. Sommerville. 1988. "HIV Testing in Glasgow Genito-Urinary Medicine Clinics, 1985–1987." *Scottish Medical Journal* 33 (4): 294–95.

Kaspar, B. 1989. "Women and AIDS: A Psychosocial Perspective." *Affilia* 4 (4): 2–22.

Kegeles, S. M., et al. 1990. "Many People Who Seek Anonymous HIV Antibody Testing Would Avoid It Under Other Circumstances." *AIDS* 4: 585–88.

Kelly, G. F. 1974. "Bisexuality and the Youth Culture." *Homosexuality Counseling Journal* 1: 16–25.

Kinsey, A. C.; W. B. Pomeroy; and C. E. Martin. 1948, 1953. *Sexual Behavior in the Human Male*. Philadelphia: W. B. Saunders.

Kipke, M.; C. Boyer; and K. Hein. 1989. "An Evaluation of an AIDS Risk-Reduction Education and Skills Training (ARRES) Program for Adolescents." Paper presented at the Fifth International Conference on AIDS, Montreal.

Klassen, A. D.; C. J. Williams; and E. E. Levitt. 1989. *Sex and Morality in the U.S.* Middletown, Conn.: Wesleyan University Press.

Klein, F. 1978. *The Bisexual Option*. New York: Arbor House.

———; B. Sepekoff; and T. J. Wolf. 1985. "Sexual Orientation: A Multi-Variable Dynamic Process." *Journal of Homosexuality* 11 (1 and 2): 35–49.

Knight, R. G. 1983. "Female Homosexuality and the Custody of Children." *New Zealand Journal of Psychology* 12 (1): 34–36.

Kolby, P., et al. 1986. "The LAV/HTLV-III Screening in Copenhagen. Epidemiological Results from Four Clinics over the Period 1 July 1984 to 1 April 1985." *Danish Medical Bulletin* 33 (5): 268–70.

Kreiss, J. K., et al. 1986. "AIDS Virus Infection in Nairobi Prostitutes." *New England Journal of Medicine* 314 (7): 414–18.

Kroef, Justus M. van der. 1954. "Transvestism and the Religious Hermaphrodite in Indonesia." *University of Manila Journal of East Asiatic Studies* 3:3 (April): 257–65.

Kulick, D. 1985. "Homosexual Behavior, Culture, and Gender in Papua, New Guinea." *Ethnos* 7–2: 15.

Kumar, B., and M. W. Ross. 1990. *Homosexual Behavior and HIV Infection Risks in Indian Males: A Cross-Cultural Comparison*.

Lancaster, R. N. 1988. "Subject Honor and Object Shame: The Cochon and the Milieu-Specific Construction of Stigma and Sexuality in Nicaragua." *Ethnology* 27: 111–25.

Leventhal, H. 1973. "Changing Attitudes and Habits to Reduce Risk Factors in Chronic Disease." *American Journal of Cardiology* 31: 57–80.

———; J. C. Watts; and F. Pagano. 1967. "Effects of Fear and Instructions on How to Cope with Danger." *Journal of Personality and Social Psychology* 6: 313–21.

Lever, J. 1989. "Behavioral Patterns of Bisexual Males in the U.S., 1982." Paper presented at the CDC Workshop on Bisexuality and AIDS, Atlanta, Ga.

———; W. Rogers; S. P. Carson; R. Hertz; and D. Kanouse. 1989. "Behavioral Patterns in Bisexual Men in the U.S. in 1982." Paper presented at the Fifth International Conference on AIDS, Montreal.

Levy, R. I. 1970. "The Community Function of Tahitian Male Transvestism: A Hypothesis." Paper presented at the 126th Annual Meeting of the American Psychiatric Association, San Francisco.

Lewis, H. 1987. "Young Women's Reproductive Health Survey." *New Zealand Journal of Medicine* 100: 490–92.

London Bisexual Collective. 1988. *Bisexual Lives.* London: Off Pink Publishing.

Lord, D. J. 1980. "Human Sexuality: A Survey of the Sexual Experience of Medical Students, University of Otago." *New Zealand Medical Journal* 91: 303–305.

McCormick, A., et al. 1987. "Surveillance of AIDS in the U.K." *British Medical Journal* 295: 1466–69.

MacDonald, A. 1981. "Bisexuality: Some Comments on Research and Theory." *Journal of Homosexuality* 6 (3): 21–36.

MacFarlane, D. F. 1984. "Transsexual Prostitution in New Zealand. Predominance of Persons of Maori Extraction." *Archives of Sexual Behavior* 13 (4): 301–309.

MacNamara, D. 1965. "Male Prostitution in American Cities: Socio-Economic or Pathological Phenomenon?" *U.S. Journal of Orthopsychiatry* 35: 204.

Magaña, J. R., and J. M. Carrier. 1988. "HIV Seroprevalence and the Sexual Behavior of Mexican Farm Workers in the State of California." Paper presented at the First International Symposium on AIDS, Ixtapa, Mexico.

Magaña, J. R., et al. N.d. "A Pedagogy for Health: AIDS Education and Empowerment." Unpublished manuscript.

Maiman, L. A., and M. H. Becker. 1974. "The Health Belief Model: Origins and Correlates in Psychological Theory. *Health Education Monographs* 2: 336–53.

Manshur, M. I. Aly, and Noer Iskandar Al-Barsany. 1981. *Waria dan pengubahan kelamin ditinjau dari hukum Islam [Warias and Sex Change from the Point of View of Islamic Law]*. Yogyakarta: Nur Cahaya.

Marin, B. 1991. "Drug Abuse Treatment for Hispanics: A Culturally Appropriate Community-Oriented Approach." In *Drug and Alcohol Abuse Prevention*, R. R. Watson, ed. Clifton, N.J.: Humana Press.

Marin, B. V., and G. Marin, 1990. "Effects of Acculturation on Knowledge of AIDS and HIV Among Hispanics." *Hispanic Journal of Behavioral Sciences* 12: 110–21.

———; G. Marin; and R. Juarez. 1990. "Differences between Hispanics and Non-Hispanics in Willingness to Provide AIDS Prevention Advice." *Hispanic Journal of Behavioral Sciences* 12: 153–64.

Marin, G., and B. V. Marin. 1990. "Perceived Credibility of Channels and Sources of AIDS Information Among Hispanics." *AIDS Education and Prevention* 2: 156–63.

Marmor, M., et al. 1990. "Sex, Drugs, and HIV Infection in a New York City Hospital Outpatient Population." *Journal of Acquired Immune Symdromos* 3: 307–18.

Marshall, K. 1990. "Knowledge of AIDS and Sexual Behavior Change in a Sample of Gay Men." M.A. thesis, Victoria University, Wellington, New Zealand.

Martin, A. D., and E. S. Hetrick. 1988. "The Stigmatization of the Gay and Lesbian Adolescent." *Journal of Homsexuality* 17: 163–83.

Millan, G., and M. W. Ross. 1987. "AIDS and Gay Youth: Attitudes and Lifestyle Modifications in Young Male Homosexuals." *Community Health Studies* 11: 50–53.

Miller, J. 1982. "People, Berdaches, and Left-Handed Vicars: Human Variation in Native America." *Journal of Anthropological Research* 38: 279.

Miner, H. M., and G. de Vos. 1960. "Oasis and Casbah. Algerian Culture and Personality in Change." *Anthropological Papers* 15, Museum of Anthropology, University of Michigan.

Mishaan, C. 1985. "The Bisexual Scene in New York City." In *Bisexualities: Theory and Research*, F. Klein and T. Wolf, eds. New York: Haworth Press.

Moerkerk, H. 1987. "Educating the Community." Paper presented at the Third International Conference on AIDS, and published by the Health Education Center of Amsterdam.

————. 1988. "AIDS Prevention for Gay and Bisexual Men in Holland." Paper presented at the International Conference on Health Education, Houston, and published by the Health Education Center of Amsterdam.

Moerthiko. N.d. *Kehidupan transexual & waria* [*The Life of Transsexuals and Warias*]. Solo: Surya Murthi.

Moodie, T. D.; V. Ndatsche; and B. Sibaye. 1988. "Migrancy and Male Sexuality on the South African Gold Mines." *Journal of South African Studies* 14 (2).

Morgan, Thomas R.; M. A. Plant; and D. I. Sales. 1989. "Risks of AIDS Among Workers in the 'Sex Industry': Some Initial Results from a Scottish Study." *BMJ* 299: 148–49.

Morrow, G. D. 1989. "Bisexuality: An Exploratory Review." *Annals of Sex Research* 2: 283–306.

Nacci, P. L., and T. R. Kane. 1983. "Incidence of Sex and Sexual Aggression in Prisons." *Federal Probation* (USA) 47 (4): 21–26.

Nakra, B. R. S.; N. N. Wig; and V. K. Verma. 1978. "Sexual Behavior in the Adult North Indian Male" (A Study of 150 Patients of Male Potency Disorders). *Indian Journal of Psychiatry* 20: 118–82.

Nanda, S. 1986. "The Hijras of India: Cultural and Individual Dimensions of an Institutionalized Third Gender Role." *Journal of Homosexuality* 11 (3 and 4): 35–54.

Narain, J. P., et al. 1989. "Epidemiology of AIDS and HIV Infection in the Caribbean." *PAHO Bulletin* 23 (1 and 2): 42–49.

Oetomo, Dédé. 1988. "Tinjauan kenyataan seksologi sosial manifestasi perilaku hemoseksual di Indonesia" [A Socio-Sexological Survey of Manifestations of Homosexual Behavior in Indonesia]. In *Manifestasi homoseksual dan kenyataan dalam lingkungan sosial-budaya* [*The Reality of Homosexual Manifestations in Socio-Cultural Context*], H. Soeharno et al., eds. Surabaya: Laboratorium Biomedik, Fakultas Kedoktevan, University of Airlangga.

O'Reilly, K., and S. Aral. 1985. "Adolescence and Sexual Behavior: Trends and Implications for STD." *Journal of Adolescent Health Care* 6: 262–70.

Padian, N. 1988. "Heterosexuals and AIDS: What Is the Risk?" *Focus* 3 (3): 1.

————. 1989. "Female Partners of Bisexual Men." Paper presented at the CDC Workshop on Bisexuality and AIDS.

————, et al. 1987. "Male to Female Transmission of Human Immuno-Deficiency Virus." *Journal of the American Medical Association* 258 (6): 788–90.

Palacios, M., et al. 1990. "Ethnographic Study of Homosexual Practices in Men from Mexico." Paper presented at the Sixth International Conference on AIDS, San Francisco.

Palmer, W. 1989. "Accessing, Educating, and Researching Married Homosexual and Bisexual Men." Paper presented at the Fifth International Conference on AIDS, Montreal.

Parker, R. 1985. "Masculinity, Femininity, and Homosexuality." *Journal of Homosexuality* 11: 155–64.

————. 1987. "Acquired Immunodeficiency Syndrome in Urban Brazil." *Medical Anthropology Quarterly* 1 (2): 155–75.

————. 1988. "Sexual Culture and AIDS Education in Urban Brazil." In *AIDS 1988: AAAS Symposia Papers*. Ruth Kulstad, ed. Pp. 169–73. Washington, D.C.: American Association for the Advancement of Science.

————. 1989. "Youth, Identity, and Homosexuality: The Changing Shape of Sexual Life in Brazil." *Journal of Homsexuality* 17 (1 and 2): 267–87.

————. 1990a. *Bodies, Pleasures, and Passions: Sexual Culture in Contemporary Brazil.* Boston: Beacon Press.

————. 1990b. "Responding to AIDS in Brazil." In *Action on AIDS: National Policies in Comparative Perspective*, David Moss and Barbara Misztal, eds. Westport, Conn.: Greenwood Press.

Parkinson, P., and T. Hughes. 1987. "The Gay Community and the Response to AIDS in New Zealand." *New Zealand Medical Journal* 100: 77–79.

Paroski, P., Jr. 1987. "Health Care Delivery and the Concerns of Gay and Lesbian Adolescents." *Journal of Adolescent Health Care* 8: 188–92.

Paul, J. P. 1984. "The Bisexual Identity: An Idea without Social Recognition." *Journal of Homosexuality* 9: 45–63.

———. 1985. "Bisexuality: Reassessing Our Paradigms." *Journal of Homosexuality* 11 (1 and 2): 21–34.

Pela, A. O., and J. J. Platt. 1989. "AIDS in Africa: Emerging Trends." *Social Science and Medicine* 28 (1): 1–8.

Peristiany, J. G., ed. 1965. *Honor and Shame: The Values of Mediterranean Society.* Athens

Peterson, J. 1989. "Dangerous Liaisons: Risky Sexual Behaviors and Predictors Among Black Bisexual Men in the San Francisco Bay Area." Paper presented at the CDC Workshop on Bisexuality and AIDS, Atlanta, Ga.

———, and G. Marin. 1988. "Issues in the Prevention of AIDS Among Black and Hispanic Men." *American Psychologist* 43: 871–75.

———, et al. 1989. "Close Encounters of an Unsafe Kind: Risky Sexual Behaviors and Predictors Among Black and Hispanic Men." Paper presented at the Fifth International Conference on AIDS, Montreal.

Pinel, A. 1989. "Sexual Behavior Survey of Brazilian Men That Are Clients of Transvestite Prostitutes." Paper presented at the Fifth International Conference on AIDS, Montreal.

Piot, P., et al. 1988. "An International Perspective on AIDS." In *AIDS 1988: AAAS Symposia Papers*, Ruth Kulstad, ed. Pp. 3–18. Washington, D.C.: American Association for the Advancement of Science.

———; M. Laga; R. Ryder; and M. Chamberland. 1989. "Heterosexual Transmission of HIV." *Current Topics of AIDS* 2:11–32.

Plummer, K. 1988. "Lesbian and Gay Youth in England." *Journal of Homosexuality* 17: 195–223.

Prime People 13, no. 17 (September 23–29, 1988): 15.

Reinisch, J. 1989. Paper presented at the Fifth International Conference on AIDS, Montreal.

Remafedi, G. 1987a. "Adolescent Homosexuality." *Pediatrics* 79: 331–37.

———. 1987b. "Male Homosexuality: The Adolescent's Perspective." *Pediatrics* 79: 326–30.

Rigg, C. A. 1982. "Homosexuality in Adolescence." *Pediatric Annals* 11:10: 826–31.

Rodrigues, L., and P. Chequer. 1989. "AIDS in Brazil." *PAHO Bulletin* 23 (1–2): 30–34.

Roesler, T. A., and R. W. Deisher. 1972. "Youthful Male Homosexuality." *Journal of the American Medical Association* 219: 1018–23.

Rogers, E. 1983. *Diffusion of Innovation*. New York: Arno Press.

Ross, M. W. 1978. "The Relationship of Perceived Societal Hostility, Conformity, and Psychological Adjustment in Homosexual Men." *Journal of Homosexuality* 4: 157–68.

————. 1982. "Some Effects of Heterosexual Marriage on Homosexual Desire." *Australian Journal of Sex, Marriage, and Family* 3 (1): 25–29.

Ross, M. W. 1983. *The Married Homosexual Man*. London: Routledge & Kegan Paul.

————. 1987. "A Theory of Normal Homosexuality." In *Male and Female Homosexuality: Psychological Approaches*, L. Diamant, ed. Washington, D.C. Hemisphere.

————. 1988. "Gay Youth in Four Cultures: A Comparative Study." *Journal of Homosexuality* 17: 299–314.

————. 1988a. "Prevalence of Rise Factors for Human Immunodeficiency Virus Infection in the Australian Population." *Medical Journal of Australia* 149: 362–65.

————. 1988b. "Prevalence of Classes at Risk Behaviors for HIV Infection in a Randomly Selected Australian Population." *Journal of Sex Research* 25: 441–50.

————. 1989. "Global Patterns of Bisexuality." Paper read at WHO/ GPA/SBR—Gay and Lesbian Studies Experiment of the University of Utrecht Meeting on Bisexuality and AIDS.

————; L. J. Rogers; and H. McCulloch. 1978. "Stigma, Sex, and Society: A New Look at Gender Differentiation and Sexual Variation." *Journal of Homosexuality* 3: 315–30.

————; B. Freedman; and R. Brew. 1989. "Changes in Sexual Behavior between 1986 and 1988 in Matched Samples of Homosexually Active Men." *Community Health Studies* 13: 276–80.

————; A. D. Wodak; J. Gold; and M. Miller. N.d. "Differences across Sexual Orientation on HIV Risk Behaviors in Injecting-Drug Users." Unpublished manuscript.

Rosser, S. 1988a. "HIV Testing and Sexual Behavior in New Zealand Homosexuals." *New Zealand Journal of Medicine* 101: 493.

————. 1988b. "Auckland Homosexual Males and AIDS Prevention: A Behavioral and Demographic Description." *Community Health Studies* 12 (3): 328–38.

Rotheram-Borus, M. J., and C. Koopman. 1989. "Sexual Risk Behavior, AIDS Knowledge, and Beliefs about AIDS Among Heterosexual Runaway and Gay Male Adolescents." Unpublished manuscript.

———; C. Koopman; C. Haigere; and H. Bird. 1989. "Adolescent AIDS Awareness." Paper presented at the Annual Meeting of Child and Adolescent Psychiatry, New York.

Roumelioutou-Karayannis, A., et al. 1988. "Heterosexual Transmission of HIV in Greece." *AIDS—Research into Human Retroviruses* 4 (3): 233–36.

Rubenstein, M., and C. Slater. 1985. "A Profile of the San Francisco Bisexual Center." In *Bisexualities: Theory and Research*, F. Klein and T. Wolf, eds. New York: Haworth Press.

Sagarin, E. 1976. "Prison Homosexuality and Its Effect on Post-Prison Sexual Behavior." *Psychiatry* 39: 245–57.

Saghir, M., and E. Robins. 1973. *Male and Female Homosexuality: A Comprehensive Investigation*. Baltimore: William & Wilkins.

Sakondhavat, C., et al. 1988. "KAP Study on Sex Reproduction and Contraception in Thai Teenagers." *Medical Association of Thailand* 27 (12).

Sandfort, Th. G. M. 1982. *The Sexual Aspect of Paedophile Relations: The Experience of Twenty-Five Boys*. Amsterdam: Pan/Spartacus.

———. 1987. *Boys on Their Contracts with Men*. Elmhurst, N.Y.: Global Academic Press.

———. 1988. *Het belang van de ervaring. Over seksuele contacten in vroege jeugdjaren en seksuele gedrag en beleven op latere leeftijd*. Utrecht: Homostudies.

———. 1991. "The Argument for Adult-Child Sexual Contact. A Critical Appraisal and New Data." In *The Sexual Abuse of Children: Theory, Research, and Therapy*, W. O. Donohue and J. Geer, eds. Hillsdale, N.J.: Lawrence Erlbaum Associates.

Scacco, A. M. 1975. *Rape in Prison*. Springfield, Ill.: Charles C. Thomas.

Schwartz, P. 1989. "Bisexuality: Issues for the Study of AIDS." Paper presented at the CDC Workshop on Bisexuality and AIDS, Atlanta, Ga.

Selik, R.; K. Castro; and M. Pappaioanou. 1988. "Racial/Ethnic Differences in the Risk of AIDS in the United States." *American Journal of Public Health* 79: 1539–45.

Shah, J. M. 1961. "India and Pakistan, Sex Life." Vol. 1 of *The Encyclopedia of Sexual Behavior*, A. Ellis and A. Abarbanel, eds. New York: Hawthorn Books, Inc.

Sharma, S. K. 1989. *Hijras: The Labelled Deviants*. New Delhi: Gian Publishing House.

Shepherd, G. 1987. "Rank, Genders & Homosexuality: Mombasa as a Key to Understanding Sexual Options." In *The Cultural Construction of Homosexuality*. London: Tavistock Publications.

Shilts, R. 1989. Personal conversation.

Shrivastava, R. S.; S. Khanna; and S. M. Channabasavanna. 1985. "Transsexualism in India." *Indian Journal of Psychiatry* 27: 249–52.

Singer, M. et al. 1990. "SIDA: The Economic, Social, and Cultural Context of AIDS Among Latinos." *Medical Anthropology Quarterly* 4: 72–114.

Sinha, T. C. 1966. "The Psyche of the Garos: Anthropological Survey of India, Calcutta."

Sion, F. S., et al. 1989. "Anal Intercourse: A Risk Factor for HIV Infection in Female Partners of Bisexual Men, Rio de Janeiro, Brazil." Paper presented at the Fifth International Conference on AIDS, Montreal.

Sittitrai, W., et al. 1989. "Demographics and Sexual Practices of Male Bar Workers in Bangkok." Paper presented at the Fifth International Conference on AIDS, Montreal.

———, et al. 1990. "LIfe, Perception, and Environment Concerning Risk for HIV Infection Among Workers in Bangkok Slums." Program on AIDS, Thai Red Cross Society and Foster Parents Plan International.

———, and J. Barry. 1991. "Human Sexuality in Pattern III Countries." International Development Research Center, Canada.

Smith, G. L. 1987. "Bisexuality, A Risk Factor for HIV Infection in Military Men." *The Lancet* 2: 1402–1403.

Somasundaram, O. 1986. "Sexuality in Thirukural: The Great Tamil Book of Ethics." *Indian Journal of Psychiatry* 28: 83–86.

Sorenson, R. C. 1973. *Adolescent Sexuality in Contemporary America*. New York: World Publishing.

Soskolne, C.; R. Coates; and A. Sears. 1986. "Characteristics of a Male Homosexual/Bisexual Study Population in Toronto, Canada." *Canadian Journal of Public Health* 77: 12–16.

Stall, R., et al. 1986. "Alcohol and Drug Use During Sexual Activities and Compliance with Safe-Sex Guidelines for AIDS: The AIDS Behavioral Research Project." *Health Education Quarterly* 13: 359–71.

Standing, H., and M Kisekka. 1989. *Sexual Behavior in Sub-Saharan Africa: A Review and Annotated Bibliography*. London: Overseas Development Organization.

Strategy Research Corporation. 1989. *U.S. Hispanic Market*. Miami, Fla.

Sundet, J; I. Kvalem; P. Magnus; and I. Bakketeig. 1988. "Prevalence of Risk-Prone Sexual Behavior in the General Population of Norway." In *The Global Impact of AIDS*, A. Herring et al., eds. New York: Allen & Liss.

Taylor, C. 1985. "Mexican Male Homosexual Interaction in Public Contexts." *Journal of Homosexuality* 11 (3 and 4):117–36.

Thayer, J. 1980. "The Berdache of the Northern Plains: A Socio-Religious Perspective." *Journal of Anthropological Reserach* 36:287.

Tielman, R. A. P., and S. Polter. 1986. *Data from the National Cohort of Gay Men, First Wave*. Utrecht: Homostudies.

Troiden, R. R. 1989. "Homosexual Identity Development." *Journal of Adolescent Health Care* 9: 105–13.

Troutman, A., and J. Y. Hall. 1989. "Sex, Drugs, and AIDS: Two Innovative Appproaches to HIV/AIDS Prevention, Education, and Outreach for Minority Adolescents." Paper presented at the Fifth International Conference on AIDS, Montreal.

Umaru, Richard. 1987. " 'An Age-Long Affair.' Nigeria's Homosexuals: The Gay Culture Arrives: Cover Story." *The African Guardian*, May 14, p. 9.

University of Otago, Dunedin. 1990. *AIDS—New Zealand* 4 (February).

U.S. Bureau of the Census, 1983. *1980 Census of U.S. Population and Housing*. Washington, D.C.: Government Printing Office.

Valdespino, G., et al. 1989. AIDS in Mexico: Trends and Projections." *PAHO Bulletin* 23 (1 and 2): 20–23.

Valdespino J. L., et al. 1988. "Patrones y predicciones epidemiológicos del SIDA en México." *Sal Pub. Mex.* 30 (4): 567–93.

Van Naerssen, A. X., and K. M. G. Schreurs. 1991. "Research on Homosexuality in the Netherlands 1980–1990." *Tijdschrift voor Seksuologie*. Forthcoming.

Van Zessen, G., and Th. G. M. Sandfort. 1991. Seks en AIDS in Nederland. Den Hag: Staatsuitgeverij.

———. *Seksualiteit in Nederland. Seksueelgedrag-risico en verspreiding van AIDS.* Amsterdam: Swets & Zeitlinger.

Veugelers, P. J., et al. 1991. "Seksuele voorkeur en gedrag van Amsterdamse mannen." *Tijdschrift voor Sociale Gezondheidszorg.* Submitted for publication.

Warwick, I., and P. Aggleton. 1990. "Adolescents, Young People, and AIDS Research." In *AIDS: Individual, Cultural, and Policy Dimensions*, P. Aggleton, D. Davies, and G. Hart, eds. London: Farmer.

Weinberg, M., and C. Williams. 1974. *Male Homosexuals: Their Problems and Adaptation.* New York: Oxford University Press.

Welch, J., et al. 1986. "Willingness of Homosexual and Bisexual Men in London to Be Screened for Human Immuno-Deficiency Virus." *British Medical Journal* 293 (6552): 924.

Whitehead, H. 1981. "The Bow and the Burden Strap: A New Look at Institutionalized Homosexuality in Native North America." *In Sexual Meanings*, H. Whitehead and S. Ortner, eds. London: Cambridge Univeristy Press.

WHO Director-General. 1990. *Global Strategy for the Prevention and Control of AIDS.* Report to the 43rd World Health Assembly, WHO Headquarters (A43/6).

WHO European Region. 1989. *AIDS Policies and Programmes in the European Region.* Copenhagen: WHO CICP/GPA/O4O.

Wikan, U. 1977. "Man Becomes Woman: Transsexualism in Oman as a Key to Gender Roles." *Man* 1977: 305–19.

Wilkie, T. 1990. "Sex Survey Gives Hope for Curbing AIDS Spread." *The Independent*, February 20.

Williams, M. L. 1990. "A Model of the Sexual Relations of Young IV Drug Users." *Journal of Acquired Immune Deficiency Syndromes* 3: 192.

Witte, B. S. 1969. "Homoseksualiteit." In *Sex in Nederland*, J. D. Neerdhoff et al., eds. Utrecht: Het Spectrum.

Wolf, T. 1985. "Marriage of Bisexual Men." In *Bisexualities: Theory and Research*, F. Klein and T. Wolf, eds. New York: Haworth Press.

Wooden, W. S., and J. Parker. 1982. *Men Behind Bars: Sexual Exploitation in Prison*. New York and London: Plenum Press.

Zabin, L. S.; J. B. Hardy; E. A. Smith; and M. B. Hirsch. 1986. "Substance Use and Its Relation to Sexual Activity Among Inner-City Adolescents." *Journal of Adolescent Health Care* 7: 320–31.

Zinik, G. 1985. "Identity Conflict or Adaptive Flexibility? Bisexuality Reconsidered." *Journal of Homosexuality* 11 (1 and 2): 7–19.

Select Bibliography

Blumstein P. W., and P. Schwartz. 1977. "Bisexuality in Men." *Urban Life* 5 (3): 339–58.

Bozett, F. W. 1981. "Gay Fathers: Evolution of the Gay-Father Identity." *American Journal of Orthopsychiatry* 51 (3): 552–59.

———. 1982. "Heterogenous Couples in Heterosexual Marriages: Gay Men and Straight Women." *Journal of Marital and Family Therapy* 8: 81–89.

Brandes, S. 1981. "Like Wounded Stags: Male Sexual Ideology in an Andalusian Town." In *Sexual Meanings,* H. Whitehead and S. Ortner, eds. London: Cambridge University Press.

Braslow, C. A.; S. Safyer; and M. D. Cohen. 1983. "Screening Adolescent Male Detainees." *American Journal of Public Health* 79 (7): 902–903.

Brownfain J. J. 1985. "A Study of the Married Bisexual Male: Paradox and Resolution." *Journal of Homosexuality* 12 (1 and 2): 173–87.

Caplan, P., ed. 1987. *The Cultural Construction of Sexuality.* London: Tavistock Press.

Cates J. A. 1989. "Adolescent Male Prostitution." *Child and Adolescent Social Work* 6 (2): 151–56.

Caukins, N. R. 1974. "Male Prostitution: A Psychosocial View of Behavior." *American Journal of Orthopsychiatry* 44: 782–85.

Coleman, E. 1982. "Bisexual and Gay Men in Heterosexual Marriage: Conflicts and Resolutions in Therapy." In *Homosexuality and Psychotherapy.* Pp. 93–103. New York: Haworth Press.

———. 1985. "Integration of Male Bisexuality and Marriage." *Journal of Homosexuality* 12 (1 and 2): 189–207.

———. 1989. "The Development of Male Prostitution Activity Among Gay and Bisexual Adolescents." *Gay and Lesbian Youth.* Journal of Homosexuality series, vol. 17, nos. 1–4: 131–49.

Day, S. 1988. "Prostitute Women and AIDS: Anthropology" [editorial review]. *AIDS* 2: 421–28.

De Cecco, J. P., and M. G. Shively. 1981. "Bisexuality: Some Comments on Research and Theory." *Journal of Homosexuality* 6(3): 21–36.

Department of Health and Social Security. 1987. *AIDS: Monitoring Response to the Public Education Campaign February 1986–February 1987.* London: HMSO.

Dixon, D. 1985. "Perceived Sexual Satisfaction and Marital Happiness of Bisexual and Heterosexual Swinging Husbands." In *Bisexualities: Theory and Research,* F. Klein and T. Wolf, eds. Pp. 209–22. New York: Haworth Press.

Falola, Toyin. 1984. "Prostitution in Ibadan, 1895–1950." *The Journal of Business and Social Studies* 6, no. 2: 40–54.

Feldman, D. A., et al. 1987. "Public Awareness of AIDS in Rwanda." *Social Science and Medicine* 2(2):97–100.

Fulford, K. W., et al. 1983. "Social and Psychological Factors in the Distribution of STD in Male Attenders." *British Journal of Venereal Diseases* 59(6): 386–93.

Gachuchi, J. Mugo. 1973. "Anatomy of Prostitutes and Prostitution in Kenya." Institute of Development Studies, University of Nairobi, Working Paper No. 113: 5–6.

Gochros, J. S. 1985. "Wives' Reaction on Learning That Their Husbands Are Bisexual." *Journal of Homosexuality* 12 (1 and 2): 101–13.

Herdt, G. 1989. "Gay and Lesbian Youth, Emergent Identities and Cultural Scenes at Home and Abroad." *Journal of Homosexuality* 17 (1 and 2): 1–41.

Kurdek, L. A., and J. P. Schmitt. 1986. "Interaction of Sex Role Self-Concept with Relationship Quality and Relationship Beliefs in Married, Heterosexual Cohabiting, Gay and Lesbian Couples." *Journal of Personality and Social Psychology* 51(2): 365–70.

———. 1987. "Partner Homogamy in Married Heterosexual Cohabiting, Gay and Lesbian Couples." *Journal of Sex Research* 23(2): 212–32.

Latham, J. D., and G. D. White. 1978. "Coping with Homosexual Expression within Heterosexual Marriages: Five Case Studies." *Journal of Sex and Marital Therapy* 4(3): 198–212.

Luckenbill, D. F. 1985. "Entering Male Prostitution." *Urban Life* 14(2): 132–53.

———. 1986. "Deviant Career Mobility: The Case of Male Prostitutes." *Social Problems* 33(4): 283–96.

McManus, T. J., and M. McEvoy. 1987. "Some Aspects of Male Homosexual Behavior in the U.K." *British Journal of Sexual Medicine* 20: 110–20.

Malone, J. 1980. *Straight Women/Gay Men: A Special Relationship.* New York: The Dill Press.

Matteson, D. R. 1985. "Bisexual Men in Marriage: Is a Positive Homosexual Identity and Stable Marriage Possible?" In *Bisexualities: Theory and Research,* F. Klein and T. Wolf, eds. New York: Haworth Press.

Money, J., and C. Bohmer. 1980. "Prison Sexology: Two Personal Accounts of Masturbation, Homosexuality, and Rape." *Journal of Sex Research* 16(3): 258–66.

Morgan, T. R.; M. A. Plant; M. L. Plant; and D. I. Sales. 1989. "Risks of AIDS Among Workers in the 'Sex Industry': Some Initial Results from a Scottish Study." *British Medical Journal* 299: 148–49.

Nahas, R., and M. Turley. 1979. *The New Couple: Women and Gay Men.* New York: Seaview Books.

Pinel, A. 1989. "Sexuality Research in Brazil." Abstract ThGO10. Fifth International Conference on AIDS, Montreal.

Price, V.; B. Scanlon; and M. J. Janus. 1984. "Social Characteristics of Adolescent Male Prostitutes." *Victimology* 9(2): 211–21.

Quinn, T.; T. Zacharuas; and R. St. John. 1989. "AIDS in the Americas: An Emerging Public Crisis." *New England Journal of Medicine* 320: 1005–7.

Radcliffe-Brown, A. R., and Daryll Forde, eds. 1950. *African Systems of Kinship and Marriage.* London: International Africans Institute, Oxford University.

Ratnam, K. V. 1985. "Awareness of AIDS Among Transsexual Prostitutes in Singapore." *Singapore Medical Journal*: 519–21.

Ross, L. H. 1971. "Modes of Adjustment of Married Homosexuals." *Social Problems* 18: 385–93.

Ross, M. W. 1979. "Bisexuality: Fact or Fallacy?" *British Journal of Sexual Medicine* (February): 49–50.

———. 1989. "Global Patterns of Bisexuality." Paper presented at World Health Organization/University of Utrecht Meeting on Bisexuality and HIV/AIDS.

Sion, F. S. 1988. "The Importance of Anal Intercourse in Transmission of HIV to Women." Paper read at the Fourth International Conference on AIDS, Stockholm.

Weeks, J. 1981. *Sex, Politics, and Society: The Regulation of Sexuality since 1800*. Harlow: Longman.

———. 1982. "Inverts, Perverts, and Mary-Annes: Male Prostitution and the Regulation of Homosexuality in England and Wales in the Nineteenth and Early Twentieth Centuries." *Journal of Homosexuality* 5: 113–34.

———. 1985. *Sexuality and its Discontents*. London: Routledge and Kegan Paul.

Williams, W. L. 1986. "Persistence and Change in the Berdache Tradition Among Contemporary Lakota Indians." *Journal of Homosexuality* 11(3 and 4): 191–200.

Winkleskin, W., Jr.; J. A. Wiley; N. Padian; and J. Leg. 1986. "Potential for Transmission of AIDS–associated Retrovirus from Bisexual Males in San Francisco to Their Female Sexual Contacts." *Journal of the American Medical Association* 255(7): 901.

Wolf, T. J. 1987. "Group Counseling for Bisexual Men." *Journal for Specialists in Group Work* (November 1987): 162–65.

Index of Contributors

Tade Akin Aina, Ph.D. is a senior lecturer in the field of sociology at the University of Lagos in Nigeria. He received his doctorate in sociology.

Mary Boulton, Ph.D. is a lecturer in sociology as applied to medicine at St. Mary's Hospital Medical School in London. She received her doctorate in sociology from the University of London. Her research interests include communication between doctors and patients as well as health beliefs and behavior of homosexual and bisexual men in relation to HIV/AIDS.

Tim Brown, Ph.D. is assistant professor of electrical engineering at the University of Hawaii in Honolulu. He received his Ph.D. in physics from the University of Hawaii in 1984. His current fields of interest include computer modeling of HIV and STD spread, incorporation of sociocultural information into such models, and exploration of their role in public health decision making.

Manuel Carballo, Ph.D., works as the chief of the research and development program on substance abuse at the World Health Organization in Geneva, Switzerland. He was the previous head of the Social and Behavioral Research unit of WHO's Global Programme on AIDS.

Joe M. Carrier, Ph.D., is affiliated with the AIDS Community Education Project under Epidemiology and Disease Prevention at the Health Care Agency of Orange County in Santa Anna, California. He received his doctorate in anthropology from The University of California, Irvine, and has been conducting research on sexual behavior in Mexico and California. He is a reserve member of the Mental Health AIDS Research Review Committee, NIMH.

Joseph A. Catania, Ph.D. is affiliated with the Center of AIDS Prevention Studies (CAPS) at The University of California, San Francisco.

Jane Chetwynd, B.S., M.S., Ph.D., is senior lecturer in the Department of Community Health and Medicine at Christchurch School of Medicine, University of Otago, in Christchurch, New Zealand. She received her doctorate from the University of London. Her research interests include knowledge, attitudes, and behavior about HIV/AIDS, motivation for changing sexual behavior, social and sexual behavior among groups of homo-, hetero-, and bisexual men and women, and general practitioners and HIV/AIDS.

Anthony P. M. Coxon, B.A., Ph.D., is director of the ESCR Research Centre on Micro-Social Change and professor of sociology at the University of Essex in Colchester, as well as emeritus professor of sociological research methods at the University of Wales. He received his doctorate in sociology and his BA degree in sociology and philosophy at the University of Leeds. His research interests include sociology of sexual behavior, socio-epidemiology of HIV infection and sociology of homosexual lifestyles, representation of cognitive systems, and multidimensional scaling and classification.

Lynda S. Doll, Ph.D., is a research psychologist at the Division of HIV/AIDS of the Centers for Disease Control (CDC) in Atlanta, Georgia. She is principal investigator of multi-center studies of HIV-seropositive blood donors and gay and bisexual men involved in high-risk behavior.

Hans Elbers, M. A., is affiliated with the Dutch Office for Health Information and Education (GVO) in Amsterdam. He is coordinator of the steering committee on AIDS information and prevention for men with homosexual contacts in the Netherlands. He studied pedagogy at the Catholic University of Nijmegen, the Netherlands, and the University of Amsterdam.

María de Lourdes García García, M.D., M.S., is deputy director of the National Institute of Epidemiological Diagnosis and Reference in Mexico City. She graduated from the National Autonomous University of Mexico. Her special field of interest is research on epidemiology of AIDS and STDs.

Jean Schaar Gochros, Ph.D., is affiliated with the University of Hawaii at Manoa. She received her doctorate from the Graduate School of Social Work, University of Denver. She also has the title of Registered

Clinical Social Worker (RCSW). She has had over thirty years' experience in clinical practice, and has both taught and published in the areas of human sexuality, sex education, marriage and family relationships. Although she is primarily a clinician, her research on wives of gay and bisexual men was considered a landmark study.

Robert B. Hays, Ph.D., is an investigator attached to the Center for AIDS Prevention Studies (CAPS) at The University of California, San Francisco. He is director of the CAPS's project on young gay men.

Aart C. Hendriks, LL.M., M.A., is affiliated with the Gay and Lesbian Studies Department of the University of Utrecht, the Netherlands. He studied law and political science at the University of Leiden. His research interests include the human rights aspects of health legislation and AIDS policy making from a European perspective.

José Izazola, M.D., M.S., is a doctoral student affiliated with the Mexican School of Public Health. He studied at Harvard University. His special field of interest is research on the behavioral aspects related to AIDS.

Susan M. Kegeles, Ph.D., is research psychologist for the Center for AIDS Prevention Studies (CAPS) at The University of California, San Francisco.

Bhushan Kumar, Ph.D., is additional professor in dermatology and STDs at the Postgraduate Institute of Medical Education and Research in Chandigarh, India.

J. Raúl Magaña, Ph.D., is affiliated with the AIDS Community Education Project under Epidemiology and Disease Prevention at the Health Care Agency of Orange County in Santa Anna, California. He received his doctorate in anthropology from The University of California, Irvine, and was a Harvard fellow at the Harvard Graduate School of Education. He is a consultant to CDC for the AIDS campaign "America responds to AIDS" and member of the AMFAR Board of Advisers for the Educational and Behavioral Program.

Hans Moerkerk, M.A., is special advisor on international health affairs of the Ministry of Welfare, Health, and Cultural Affairs in Rijswijk, the Netherlands, and is the Executive Secretary of the Dutch National Committee on AIDS Control. He studied political and social sciences at the University of Amsterdam.

Dédé Oetomo, Ph.D., is lecturer in anthropology at FISIP University of Airlangga, Surabaya, Indonesia. He received his doctorate in anthropology and is affiliated with the Working Group for Indonesian Lesbians and Gay Men, KKLGN.

Manuel Palacios, M.D., M.S., is chief of the Department of AIDS Qualitative Epidemiological Surveillance of the National Institute of Epidemiological Diagnosis and Research in Mexico City. He studied at the National Autonomous University of Mexico. His research interests include behavioral aspects related to AIDS prevention.

Richard G. Parker, Ph.D., is professor of anthropology in the Institute of Social Medicine at the State University of Rio de Janeiro, Brazil. He received his doctorate in social-cultural anthropology from The University of California, Berkeley.

John Peterson, Ph.D., is research psychologist with The University of California, San Francisco, and Scientific Codirector of the Multicultural Inquiry and Research on AIDS (MIRA) division of the Center for AIDS Prevention Studies (CAPS) at The University of California, San Francisco. His primary research interests include psychosocial studies of AIDS high-risk behaviors among black populations.

Michael W. Ross, Ph.D., is deputy director of the National Centre in HIV Social Research, and associate professor of community medicine at the University of New South Wales in Sydney, Australia. He holds degrees in psychology, sociology, health education, and public health and medical science. He was educated at the University of Wellington, New Zealand; the Universities of Melbourne, of New South Wales, and of New England in Australia; the University of New York; and the University of Stockholm in Sweden.

Theo G. M. Sandfort, Ph.D., is research coordinator at the Gay and Lesbian Studies Department of the University of Utrecht, the Netherlands. He received his doctorate in psychology from the University of Utrecht.

Jaime Sepúlveda, M.D., Ph.D., is director of the General Directorate of Epidemiology and coordinator of the National AIDS Committee. He graduated from the School of Public Health at Harvard University. His fields of research include epidemiology on AIDS, research on behavioral aspects related to AIDS prevention, and the development of a national program for AIDS/HIV prevention.

Wiresit Sittitrai, Ph.D., is assistant professor at the Institute of Population Studies at Chulalongkorn University in Bangkok, Thailand, and deputy director of the AIDS Program of the Thai Red Cross Society. He received his Ph.D. degree in political science from the University of Hawaii in 1980. His current fields of interest include aging, family planning, human sexuality, and psychosocial aspects of AIDS and HIV.

Oussama Tawil, M.A., is a sociologist who obtained his masters degree at the American University of Beirut, Lebanon. He worked as a consultant to the World Health Organization's Global Programme on AIDS in the area of social and behavioral research related to HIV/AIDS. Areas of focus in the context of AIDS included risk behavior, bisexuality, and population movement.

Rob A. P. Tielman, Ph.D., is the chairman of the Gay and Lesbian Studies Department of the University of Utrecht in the Netherlands. He is professor in humanistic studies and president of the International Humanist and Ethical Union. He is also a member of the Dutch National Committee on AIDS Control. He received his doctorate in sociology from the University of Utrecht and wrote his dissertation on the history of homosexuality in the Netherlands.

José Valdespino, M.D., M.S., M.Ph., is director of the National Institute of Epidemiological Diagnosis and Reference in Mexico City. He received his doctorate from the Mexican School of Public Health. His special field of interest is research on epidemiology of AIDS and STDs.

Sirapone Virulrak, Ph.D., is dean of the Faculty of Fine and Applied Arts of Chulanongkorn University in Bangkok, Thailand. He received his Ph.D. degree in drama and theater from the University of Hawaii in 1980. His current fields of interest include drama, theater, folk arts, sociocultural aspects of the arts, and the cultural interpretation of behavior.